CLINICAL FOCUS SERIES

Difficult Asthma

CLINICAL FOCUS SERIES

Difficult Asthma

Editors

Liam G Heaney MD MRCP
Professor of Respiratory Medicine
School of Medicine, Dentistry and Biological Sciences
Queens University Belfast
Belfast, Northern Ireland, UK

Andrew Menzies-Gow BSc MBBS PhD FRCP
Consultant Physician in Respiratory Medicine
Royal Brompton Hospital
London, England, UK

JAYPEE BROTHERS MEDICAL PUBLISHERS (P) LTD.

New Delhi • London • Philadelphia • Panama

Jaypee Brothers Medical Publishers (P) Ltd.

Headquarters
Jaypee Brothers Medical Publishers (P) Ltd
4838/24, Ansari Road, Daryaganj
New Delhi 110 002, India
Phone: +91-11-43574357
Fax: +91-11-43574314
Email: jaypee@jaypeebrothers.com

Overseas Offices
J.P. Medical Ltd
83 Victoria Street, London
SW1H 0HW (UK)
Phone: +44-2031708910
Fax: +02-03-0086180
Email: info@jpmedpub.com

Jaypee-Highlights Medical Publishers Inc.
City of Knowledge, Bld. 237, Clayton
Panama City, Panama
Phone: + 507-301-0496
Fax: + 507-301-0499
Email: cservice@jphmedical.com

Jaypee Brothers Medical Publishers, Ltd
The Bourse
111 South Independence Mall East
Suite 835, Philadelphia, PA 19106, USA
Phone: + 267-519-9789
Email: joe.rusko@jaypeebrothers.com

Jaypee Brothers Medical Publishers (P) Ltd
17/1-B Babar Road, Block-B, Shaymali
Mohammadpur, Dhaka-1207
Bangladesh
Mobile: +08801912003485
Email: jaypeedhaka@gmail.com

Jaypee Brothers Medical Publishers (P) Ltd
Shorakhute, Kathmandu
Nepal
Phone: +00977-9841528578
Email: jaypee.nepal@gmail.com

Website: www.jaypeebrothers.com
Website: www.jaypeedigital.com

Inquiries for bulk sales may be solicited at: jaypee@jaypeebrothers.com

This book has been published in good faith that the contents provided by the contributors contained herein are original, and is intended for educational purposes only. While every effort is made to ensure the accuracy of information, the publisher and the editors specifically disclaim any damage, liability, or loss incurred, directly or indirectly, from the use or application of any of the contents of this work. If not specifically stated, all figures and tables are courtesy of the editors. Where appropriate, the readers should consult with a specialist or contact the manufacturer of the drug or device.

Clinical Focus Series
Difficult Asthma / Eds. Liam G Heaney, Andrew Menzies-Gow
First Edition: **2013**

ISBN 978-93-5090-299-8

Printed at: S. Narayan & Sons

CONTENTS

CONTRIBUTORS

EDITORS

Liam G Heaney MD MRCP
Professor of Respiratory Medicine
School of Medicine, Dentistry and Biological Sciences
Queens University Belfast
Belfast, Northern Ireland, UK

Andrew Menzies-Gow BSc MBBS PhD FRCP
Consultant Physician in Respiratory Medicine
Royal Brompton Hospital
London, England, UK

CONTRIBUTING AUTHORS

Ian M Adcock PhD FSB
Professor
Respiratory Cell and Molecular Biology
National Heart and Lung Institute
Imperial College London
London, England, UK

Christopher Brightling MRCP PhD
Wellcome Senior Clinical Fellow
Honorary Consultant
Institute for Lung Health
Leicester, England, UK

Rekha Chaudhuri MD
Associate Specialist and Honorary
Senior Clinical Lecturer
Department of Respiratory Medicine
Gartnavel General Hospital and
University of Glasgow
Glasgow, Scotland, UK

Kian F Chung MD DSc FRCP
Professor of Respiratory Medicine and
Head of Experimental Studies
National Heart and Lung Institute
Imperial College London
London, England, UK

Rob Horne BSc MSc PhD FRPharmS
Professor of Behavioural Medicine
Head of Department of Practice and
Policy
Director, Centre for Behavioural
Medicine
UCL School of Pharmacy
London, England, UK

Adel H Mansur PhD FRCP
Department of Respiratory
Birmingham Heartlands Hospital
Birmingham, England, UK

Robert Niven MBChB BSc MD MFOM FRCP
Senior Lecturer in Respiratory Medicine
The University of Manchester and
University Hospital of South Manchester
North West Lung Centre
University Hospital of South Manchester
Manchester, England, UK

Ciaran O'Neill BSc PhD
Professor of Health Technology
Assessment
Cairns School of Business and
Economics
National University of Galway
Galway, Ireland

Alison Pooler PhD MSc BSc PGCHPE
RGN RNT
School of Nursing and Midwifery
Keele University
Staffordshire, England, UK

Michael D Shields MBChB MD FRCP
FRCPCH
Professor of Child Health and
Consultant Pediatrician
Queen's University Belfast and Royal
Belfast Hospital for Sick Children
Belfast, Northern Ireland, UK

Annemarie Sykes MBBS MRCP PhD
Clinical Lecturer
Respiratory Medicine,
Imperial College London
London, England, UK

Claire Telford
Centre for Public Health
School of Medicine, Dentistry and
Biomedical Sciences
Queen's University Belfast
Belfast, Northern Ireland, UK

Surendran Thavagnanam MBBCh BAO
MD MRCPCH
Associate Professor and Consultant
Pediatrician
University Malaya and University
Malaya Medical Centre
Lembah Pantai, Kuala Lumpur,
Malaysia

Neil C Thomson MBChB MD FRCP
Professor
Institute of Infection, Immunity, and
Inflammation
University of Glasgow
Glasgow, Scotland, UK

Jennifer M Versnel BSc MSc MPhil
Business Innovation Consultant
Asthma UK
London, England, UK

Sally E Wenzel MD
Director
University of Pittsburgh Asthma
Institute
Pittsburgh, Pennsylvania, USA

PREFACE

Asthma is common and affects an estimated 300 million people worldwide. The diagnosis is often straightforward, and symptoms respond well to standard doses of inhaled therapy. However, approximately 5–10% of patients with asthma do not respond well and have poor symptomatic control, despite prescription of currently available therapies. These patients are often referred to as having "difficult asthma". This poor response to conventional therapy is not always due to underlying asthma severity. Systematic multidisciplinary approaches to clinical evaluation have sought to dissect the complexity of this clinical population and demonstrated how targeted intervention can improve outcome. Some patients do have severe refractory disease, where there is a suboptimal response to currently available therapies, and in these cases, novel therapies, including specific monoclonal antibodies against key biological targets, are becoming available.

The purpose of this book is to provide medical students, postgraduate fellows, general practitioners, and specialists a succinct, easy-to-read, well-illustrated, and comprehensive review of difficult asthma. The book brings together the opinion of international experts in the field and provides a pragmatic overview of the clinical problems, giving an insight into the complexity of this population and providing a framework for managing these patients. It covers the etiology, pathogenesis, and management of refractory asthma and novel therapeutic approaches in this group. Importantly, it gives an insight into the patient's perspective of severe asthma and the associated disproportionate use of healthcare resources and major economic burden of poorly controlled asthma.

We hope that this book will be of use not only for pulmonologists and internists but also for practitioners of other specialties, because this clinical problem is often encountered by nonpulmonologists.

Finally, we would like to record our sincere thanks to the group of international physicians and academicians who, despite their busy schedules, provided outstanding educational material for this book.

Liam G Heaney
Andrew Menzies-Gow

Acknowledgments

We would like to acknowledge the huge effort from the international experts who have contributed to this book. When approached about the project, all responded with great enthusiasm, reflecting their passion to promote understanding and improve care for patients with difficult-to-control asthma.

Our special gratitude goes to the editorial team of M/s Jaypee Brothers Medical Publishers (P) Ltd., New Delhi, India, who drove the project forward and was a great assistance throughout.

Definition, Epidemiology, and Phenotypes of Severe Asthma

Sally E Wenzel

INTRODUCTION

Asthma has long been defined by the presence of reversible airflow limitation (or bronchial hyper-responsiveness) in the setting of appropriate symptoms.[1,2] In more recent years, inflammation has loosely been connected to the definition of asthma, but in most cases no measurement or characterization of inflammation in a given clinical patient is performed. This current definition of asthma is almost certainly broad enough to encompass numerous diseases, syndromes, or phenotypes. Yet, until recently, only modest effort had been undertaken to differentiate these different patients and their "conditions." Further, in milder forms of asthma, most patients are reasonably well treated with nonspecific anti-inflammatory and bronchodilating medications and the ability to distinguish subgroups is less important. However, patients with a diagnosis of severe asthma present with a broad range of characteristics, usually in conjunction with poor response to corticosteroids (CSs) and other traditional therapies and, therefore, distinguishing one subgroup from another is likely to be clinically and scientifically important.

DEFINING SEVERE ASTHMA

Interestingly, similar to the definition of asthma, most definitions of severe asthma are also general. In addition to ruling out "difficult-to-treat asthma," most currently utilized definitions require that a patient meets the general diagnosis of asthma and then rely primarily on dependency for high-dose CS treatment in light of ongoing symptoms, frequent or severe exacerbations, and/or poor lung function. Numerous specific definitions have been proposed for severe asthma over the last 20 years, including those proposed by the European Respiratory Society (ERS) and American Thoracic Society (ATS).[3,4] Both of these earlier definitions contrasted with various guidelines-based definitions by inclusion of the need for background therapy with high-dose inhaled or systemic CS, and in the case of ERS definition, evaluation and treatment by an asthma specialist. The ATS definition went so far as to propose two major criteria and seven minor criteria encompassing aspects of treatment and control.

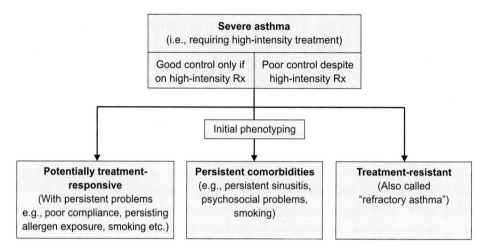

Figure 1-1 Difficult asthma, defined by poorly controlled symptoms despite treatment or controlled symptoms only on high-dose treatment can be initially subgrouped into those who are difficult to control because of potentially treatment responsive issues, persistent comorbidities, or who have truly treatment resistant (refractory) disease. *Adapted from* Taylor DR, Bateman ED, Boulet LP, et al. A new perspective on concepts of asthma severity and control. *Eur Respir J.* 2008;32:545-54.

More recently, the World Health Organization (WHO) defined severe asthma by first identifying three "global" subgroups: (i) untreated severe asthma, an enormous problem in areas of the world where current therapies for asthma are not widely available, (ii) treatment-resistant severe asthma, and (iii) difficult-to-treat (but potentially responsive) asthma.[5] Treatment-resistant asthma was further differentiated into those who achieve control on current medications and those who are never able to achieve control despite current medications (Figure 1-1).

Very recently, the Innovative Medicine Initiative (IMI) proposed the term "problematic asthma" as an umbrella term for poorly controlled asthma.[6] The consensus statement then categorized problematic asthma into two groups: "difficult asthma," a group in which the disease itself may not be severe but issues with adherence and poor treatment of confounders make it difficult to control and "severe refractory asthma," a term reserved for those who have persistent poor control, frequent exacerbations despite acceptable adherence to high-intensity treatment, and treatment of comorbidities (Table 1-1). This IMI definition of asthma will likely form the basis of future joint ATS-ERS definitions.

These definitions from WHO and IMI are based on data from recent large scale studies of severe asthma, which have greatly expanded on our understanding of the range of characteristics accompanying patients with this syndrome.[7-9] As part of these studies, the presence of frequent and/or severe exacerbations, low baseline

Table 1-1	Diagnosis of Severe Refractory Asthma—An International Consensus Statement from the Innovative Medicine Initiative

1. Requires confirmed diagnosis of asthma, compliance/adherence, and comorbidities addressed
2. All severe asthma patients require treatment with high-intensity treatment by an asthma specialist to prevent patients from becoming uncontrolled or who remain uncontrolled

Adults:

a. High-dose therapy: high-dose inhaled CS and LABA (or LT modifier)/or systemic CS. (High-dose inhaled CS-fluticasone > 1000 µg/day)

b. Uncontrolled defined as any one of the following:

   i. *Poor symptom control:* ACQ consistently > 1.5 (or "not well controlled" by published guidelines)

   ii. *Frequent or severe exacerbations*: 2 or systemic CS requiring, including those requiring ER visits or hospitalizations, per year

c. Controlled or uncontrolled asthma on these high doses of inhaled CSs or systemic CSs (or additional biologics) places a patient at high future risk for side effects from medications

CS, corticosteroid; LABA, long-acting β_2-agonist; LT, leukotriene; ACQ, Asthma Control Questionnaire; ER, emergency room.

Source: Bel EH, Sousa A, Fleming L, Bush A, Chung KF, Versnel J, et al. Diagnosis and definition of severe refractory asthma: an international consensus statement from the Innovative Medicine Initiative. *Thorax.* 2011;66:910-17.

lung function and near daily symptoms, all in the face of treatment with high doses of inhaled and/or oral CS have been identified as present in the majority of severe asthma patients.

Distinguishing Severe Asthma from Difficult-to-treat Asthma

When a patient presents with any or all of these characteristics, a physician should first determine whether a patient has severe asthma or whether the asthma is in reality, not severe, but difficult-to-treat (Figure 1-1).[5,10] This often requires evaluation, by an asthma specialist, of comorbid conditions, including those related to compliance/adherence, sinusitis, allergies, gastroesophageal reflux disease (GERD), and psychosocial issues. Studies suggest that adequately addressing these issues will improve the clinical picture in about 50% of patients.[11] However, despite the high prevalence of GERD and psychologic disturbances in asthma, particularly depression, treatment of these comorbidities appears to do little to improve asthma outcomes.[12,13] Additionally, some comorbidities, including sinusitis and obesity, can be difficult-to-treat and may contribute to the overall refractoriness of severe disease. Significant airflow limitation and air trapping, either by quantitative computed tomography (CT) imaging or physiologic measures, are also often seen in severe refractory asthma and are not easily improved.[14-16]

SEVERE ASTHMA PHENOTYPES AND THEIR EPIDEMIOLOGY

As noted, the definition of severe asthma still relies primarily on nonspecific clinical characteristics. Data from both European and North American cohorts, using both biased and unbiased approaches, now strongly support the presence of several subgroups or phenotypes of severe asthma, all of which meet the simple clinical/physiologic definitions for asthma and severe asthma noted earlier. Characterization of these phenotypes should eventually allow identification of genetic, genomic, proteomic, and lipidomic biomarkers, which better define these phenotypes.

Phenotype Definition

The concept of phenotype has been recognized and defined as observable characteristics of an organism, which develop from the interaction of the organism with its environment. In relation to asthma, multiple different terms have been used to identify phenotypes, including phenotypes related to clinical characteristic factors (severity, fixed airflow limitation, and age at onset), which associate or trigger asthma (allergy, aspirin) and finally, pathobiologic characteristics (neutrophils/eosinophils). However, as this field expands and, becomes better defined, a phenotype may better be understood as a "grouping" of several observable or measureable characteristics, often including elements from each of those categories (Table 1-2). As an example, the presence of high numbers of eosinophils in blood/sputum, when evaluated in isolation are in actuality only an observable characteristic. Recent studies are now recognizing that the presence of high numbers of lung eosinophils, especially in someone treated with CS, often has additional associated characteristics, including later age of asthma onset, frequent and severe exacerbations, sinus disease and/or nasal polyps, requirements for high doses of CS to maintain control, and in a subgroup, sensitivity to nonsteroidal anti-inflammatory.[17-21] For this chapter, only phenotypes, which satisfy the criteria for multiple consistent and reproducible characteristics from epidemiologic to genetics to biomarkers will be included (Table 1-2).

Approaches to Phenotyping

While the number and type of characteristics required to define a phenotype have not been determined, it is likely that at least 3–4 shared characteristics ranging

Table 1-2	Severe Asthma Phenotypes with Numerous Identifiable and Consistent Characteristics
• Allergic asthma (early or late onset) • Adult onset/persistent eosinophilic asthma • Aspirin sensitive asthma	• Late adult onset/female/hormonal and obesity linked • Adult onset/infection-related

from similarities in epidemiology, genetics, physiology, clinical characteristics, and responses to therapy to the presence of specific biomarkers or pathobiologic mechanisms should be present. These phenotypes can be identified using a biased approach based on observations and analysis of patients as seen clinically, or through un- or lesser-biased statistical approaches. No truly unbiased approaches to phenotyping of asthma or severe asthma have yet been published, as even the statistical cluster analyses were based on initial biased associations of certain characteristics (medication use or eosinophils for instance) and assumptions of what variables to include in the models. Intriguingly, however, both biased and unbiased approaches are pointing towards similar phenotypes and the results are complementary.

Two statistical clustering (unbiased) analyses of severe asthma have been published to date. These cluster analyses differed in their input, with the Leicester (UK) cluster not including lung function as an input variable, but including sputum eosinophils, while the Severe Asthma Research Program (SARP)/US cluster analysis included lung function, but did not include lung/sputum eosinophils.[20,22] Despite these different approaches, more similarities than differences exist. In both models, age at onset of asthma was one of the strong independent predictors of phenotype group, with younger age at onset asthma tending to associate with an allergy related process, consistent with previous biased studies, which identified early onset or "extrinsic" asthma as a primarily allergic disease with strong hereditary component and onset in early childhood.[21,23] The SARP approach identified five separate clusters, primarily differentiated by lung function, β-agonist use, and age at the onset (Figure 1-2). The Leicester approach identified four clusters, including those with early onset, primarily allergic asthma of different severities. Interestingly, both studies suggested that early onset/allergic asthma makes up about 35–40% of all severe asthmatics.

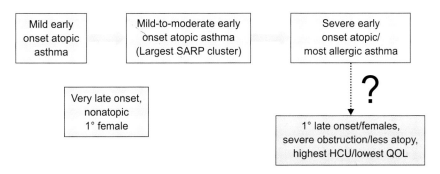

Figure 1-2 The five clusters identified by Moore et al. SARP, Severe Asthma Research Program; HCU, health care utilization; QOL, quality of life. *Adapted from* Moore WC, Meyers DA, Wenzel SE, Teague WG, Li H, Li X, et al. Identification of asthma phenotypes using cluster analysis in the Severe Asthma Research Program. *Am J Respir Crit Care Med.* 2010;181:315-23.

Both cluster analyses identified at least two different clusters of patients with later onset of disease. In each analysis, a group of late onset asthmatics were identified with symptoms out of proportion to their airway obstruction [as measured by forced expiratory volume in 1 second (FEV$_1$)% predicted in the SARP cluster]. These patients tended to be women, with very late onset (median age at onset in the 5th decade) of disease, who were likely to be obese, and in SARP, were likely to be menopausal or have undergone a surgical menopause. However, inflammatory parameters differed in the two analyses, the SARP patient cluster showing evidence for ongoing eosinophilic and neutrophilic inflammation, while the Leicester cluster had rather non-inflammatory by sputum analysis.

The Leicester cohort also identified a group of late onset, highly eosinophilic severe asthmatics who were exacerbation prone. These late onset eosinophilic asthmatics have also been identified in biased clinical studies supporting the existence of this phenotype.[21] Whether this cluster is similar to the "6th" SARP cluster, with late onset, less allergic disease is not yet clear given the differences in study design and approach.

Thus, combining biased and unbiased studies of severe asthma available to date, at least three different subgroups of severe asthma have been consistently identified, which include enough different characteristics to be termed a phenotype. These phenotypes include: (i) allergic/early onset severe asthma, (ii) late onset eosinophilic asthma despite CS therapy [with a subset of aspirin intolerant asthma (AIA)], and (iii) a less well-defined very late onset, obese, and highly symptomatic group consisting primarily of women.

However, it is clear that as our molecular understanding of severe asthma improves, our precision in defining phenotypes and associated biomarkers will also improve (Figure 1-3). It is hoped that this investment will lead to a more personalized, effective, and a safe approach to the therapy for greater numbers of severe asthmatics.

SPECIFIC SEVERE ASTHMA PHENOTYPES

Allergic Severe Asthma

From an epidemiologic perspective, this group of severe asthmatic patients primarily develop their disease in childhood well before the age of 10.[21,22] Although, allergic asthma with onset in adulthood certainly occurs, there is often a history of allergic reactions of some sort since childhood.[24] This phenotype also appears to have a strong genetic component, with a family history of asthma more common in these asthmatics than in later onset disease.[21,22] It remains unclear what percentage of these early onset severe asthma patients had severe asthma since childhood and how many progressively developed severe asthma over time. However, the available evidence suggests that more severe asthma in early childhood is more likely to be

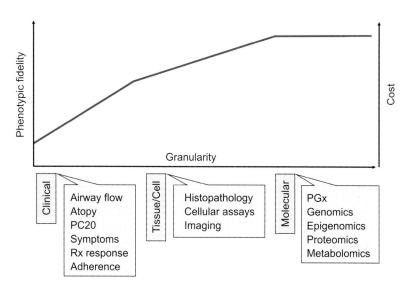

Figure 1-3 Increasing understanding of the molecular basis of severe asthma phenotypes, while initially expensive, should lead to improvements in the ability to personalize care for each phenotype. *From* Bousquet J, Mantzouranis E, Cruz AA, Aït-Khaled N, Baena-Cagnani CE, Bleecker ER, et al. Uniform definition of asthma severity, control, and exacerbations: document presented for the World Health Organization Consultation on Severe Asthma. *J Allergy Clin Immunol.* 2010;126:926-38; *with permission.*

related to more severe asthma in adulthood, with few children with mild asthma progressing to more severe asthma.[25,26] This early onset allergic group appears to constitute around 40% of all severe asthmatics. In both cluster analyses, patients in this group appeared to be at the extreme end of an allergic asthma phenotype. In the SARP cluster, these patients were more likely to be older, with a longer duration of disease, and were more likely to have reported a history of pneumonia than their milder counterparts. Severe asthmatics with this phenotype are likely to have a high number of allergic skin test reactions, a higher systemic immunoglobulin E (IgE) level, and greater environmental triggers.[21,22]

Allergy-specific therapeutic approaches have long existed. Allergy immuno-therapy in this population is not without risk and there are no data to support its ability to prevent development of severe allergic asthma. In contrast, the introduction of anti-IgE (omalizumab) for the treatment of allergic asthma was one of the 1st attempts to phenotypically direct therapy. Unfortunately, allergic asthma was defined in a rather limited way for these studies. In any case, omalizumab has shown modest efficacy in severe asthma patients with evidence for specific and elevated systemic IgE.[27] Intriguingly, however, it does not appear to work in more than 30–50% of "appropriate" patients for unclear reasons, and does not appear to have significant benefit in severe asthmatics on oral CSs.[28] Whether anti-IgE would be more effective in individuals more rigidly defined as allergic or whether understanding the immmuno-pathology around IgE would improve responder rates awaits further study.

The presence of an IgE-related process in the airways supports a Th2 immune process.[29] Proof of the importance of Th2 cytokines to severe allergic asthma is not yet present, although a recent gene expression study of mild asthma suggested that 50% of mild asthmatics manifested a Th2 gene expression profile associated with atopy/allergic disease.[30] Supporting this involvement of Th2 in mild allergic asthma are studies with a mutein of interleukin (IL)-4, which blocks the IL-4 receptor α (IL-4Rα, pitrakinra). These studies demonstrated improvement in both the late fall in FEV_1 in response to allergen challenge, as well as in levels of exhaled nitric oxide.[31,32] In very small numbers, the response to pitrakinra also appeared to have a genetic component with data suggesting that previously described risk alleles at single nucleotide polymorphisms (SNPs) in IL-4Rα were predictive of response to therapy.[32,33] In a 12-week study of a global population of patients with more severe asthma (symptomatic despite modest dose ICS), an antibody to IL-4Rα failed to show efficacy, although a modest benefit was seen in the most symptomatic subjects.[34] Unfortunately, no further attempts to characterize the "phenotype," the responders, was reported in relation to this study. Whether identification of an "allergic/Th2" phentoype would improve the response, particularly in severe asthma, will require further study. Interestingly, studies of lung inflammatory processes (sputum and to some degree tissue) have not consistently shown a predominant eosinophilic inflammation in severe early onset asthma.[21,22] In fact, the combination of eosinophilic and neutrophilic inflammation has been associated with the most severe (frequent exacerbations, symptoms, and systemic CS use) disease.[35] Whether this implies the additional importance of other immune pathways (particularly Th17) in severe allergic asthma remains to be determined.[36,37]

Late Onset Hypereosinophilic Severe Asthma (Including Aspirin Intolerant Asthma)

As noted previously, later onset asthma includes several potential phenotypes, although the hypereosinophilic phenotype is perhaps the most distinct, making up around 25% of the severe asthma group, with a recent study confirming the persistence of hypereosinophilia over time.[20,21,38] Although two later onset groups were identified in the Moore's clusters, this particular phenotype was not identified. However, it may have been a subset of the later onset, very severe cluster five.[22] Epidemiologically, these patients are generally healthy until their late 20s or beyond. An upper or lower respiratory tract infection, with or without the development of chronic sinusitis and nasal polyps can precede the onset of asthma. These individuals typically have both blood and lung eosinophils in high numbers, which persist even in the face of high-dose inhaled CSs. Both eosinophils and cysteinyl leukotrienes (cLTs) are typically higher than those seen in severe allergic asthma.[21]

A subset reports asthma worsening, often severe, in response to aspirin (Samter's triad), but this phenotype can exist without aspirin intolerance. This AIA is well known to develop later in life and is strongly associated with elevations in eosinophils and cyteinyl leukotrienes.[39,40] AIA was the first subgroup of asthma to have specific treatment trials. Because of the high cysteinyl leukotriene levels, treatment with a 5-lipoxygenase inhibitor and/or leukotriene receptor antagonist can lead to marked improvements in both lung function and clinical symptoms.[21,41,42]

Despite the success of leukotriene modifying drugs in AIA, specific treatment trials in the broader category of hypereosinophilic severe asthma have not been undertaken. However, recent studies with an antibody against the proeosionphilic/ Th2 cytokine IL-5 (mepolizumab) have successfully targeted severe asthmatics with high eosinophills.[43,44] These studies did not specifically target later onset disease; however, evaluation of the age at onset of the subjects included in the two published clinical trials suggest that the majority of subjects in the trials were later/adult onset hypereosinophilic asthma.

Pathobiologically, although these patients are generally less atopic than those with early onset disease, IgE levels can be elevated and fractional exhaled nitric oxide (FeNO) is often very high, despite inhaled CSs. These findings, combined with the improvement with antibodies against the traditionally Th2-linked cytokine IL-5 suggest that these patients are likely to have a Th2 bias as well, but further confirmation of this relationship is required.

"Later" Onset Symptom-prone Severe Asthma

While this group is included here, as it has, to some degree, been observed in both cluster analyses and is clinically recognized, information on the natural history, pathogenesis, and responses to therapy is limited. In both clusters, these patients were primarily women, with the onset of the disease in the 5th decade or later. Obesity is common and there is an association with natural or surgical menopause.[20,22] While systemic CSs in exacerbations are extremely common, more severe exacerbations requiring intensive care or mechanical ventilation rarely occur. Airway obstruction is less than in the other severe asthma phenotypes, but the duration of disease is also less. The pathobiology is unknown with the first cluster analysis suggesting a paucity of inflammation while the 2nd one suggested ongoing eosinophilic and neutrophilic inflammation. Whether targeted weight loss or hormonally based approaches would be helpful awaits further study.

Additional Potential Severe Asthma Phenotypes

While the previous three phenotypes have been consistently described and all present with several linked characteristics, it is likely that additional phenotypes exist. Possible phenotypes include those linked to an initiating upper respiratory infection, with associated chronic bronchitic or even bronchiectatic type changes linked to atypical bacteria or viruses, smoking, severe asthma, and others. Some of these later onset asthmatics appear to have a neutrophilic type of inflammation, which has been reported to respond to macrolide antibiotic therapy.[45] However, no definitive link to a specific organism has been found, suggesting the response to the macrolide could also be due to anti-inflammatory as opposed to antibiotic effects of the drug. This neutrophilic inflammation also appears to be associated with greater past/current tobacco use, neutrophil elastases, and lower lung function.[21,46] A further study of circulating neutrophil gene expression also suggested that the neutrophilic phenotype influenced genes related to cell mobility, apoptosis, and the NF-κB cascade.[47] However, targeted therapies beyond macrolide antibiotics have not been attempted.

A final phenotype bears mention as a specific treatment trial suggested efficacy of the antifungal agent itraconazole in asthmatics in the UK with fungal sensitivity.[16] Other than rather severe asthma and sensitization to one of several fungal allergens, no additional defining characteristics were observed. Thus, whether this fungal associated severe asthma is merely a subset of allergic asthma or a different phenotype, which will consistently respond better to antifungal therapy, requires further study.

CONCLUSION

Severe asthma remains a syndrome loosely defined by clinical and physiological changes, without specific biomarkers or pathobiology. Patients with severe asthma, who require current gold standard medications to achieve control, or who never achieve control represent a mix of patient phenotypes, at least three of which have been consistently recognized using both biased and unbiased approaches, and which, to some degree have had successful approaches using targeted therapy. Continued cross-sectional and more importantly, longitudinal and interventional studies are needed to refine our ability to phenotype severe asthma. Future studies, which integrate clinical, pathopysiologic, genetic, and genomic data, including confirmation using targeted biologic therapies should enhance our understanding and treatment of these difficult patients.

REFERENCES

1. National Asthma Education and Prevention Program Expert Panel Report 3: Guidelines for the Diagnosis and Management of Asthma (National Heart Lung and Blood Institutes, 2007).
2. Global Initiative for Asthma. Global Strategy for Asthma Management and Prevention – Updated 2008. Available from URL: www.ginasthma.com.
3. Proceedings of the ATS workshop on refractory asthma: current understanding, recommendations, and unanswered questions. American Thoracic Society. *Am J Respir Crit Care Med.* 2000;162:2341-51.

4. Chung KF, Godard P, Adelroth E, Ayres J, Barnes N, Barnes P, et al. Difficult/therapy-resistant asthma: the need for an integrated approach to define clinical phenotypes, evaluate risk factors, understand pathophysiology and find novel therapies. ERS Task Force on Difficult/Therapy-Resistant Asthma. European Respiratory Society. *Eur Respir J.* 1999;13:1198-208.

5. Bousquet J, Mantzouranis E, Cruz AA, Aït-Khaled N, Baena-Cagnani CE, Bleecker ER, et al. Uniform definition of asthma severity, control, and exacerbations: document presented for the World Health Organization Consultation on Severe Asthma. *J Allergy Clin Immunol.* 2010;126:926-38.

6. Bel EH, Sousa A, Fleming L, Bush A, Chung KF, Versnel J, et al. Diagnosis and definition of severe refractory asthma: an international consensus statement from the Innovative Medicine Initiative (IMI). *Thorax.* 2011;66:910-7.

7. The ENFUMOSA cross-sectional European multicentre study of the clinical phenotype of chronic severe asthma. European Network for Understanding Mechanisms of Severe Asthma. *Eur Respir J.* 2003;22:470-7.

8. Dolan CM, Fraher KE, Bleecker ER, Borish L, Chipps B, Hayden ML, et al. Design and baseline characteristics of the epidemiology and natural history of asthma: Outcomes and Treatment Regimens (TENOR) study: a large cohort of patients with severe or difficult-to-treat asthma. *Ann Allergy Asthma Immunol.* 2004;92:32-9.

9. Moore WC, Bleecker ER, Curran-Everett D, Erzurum SC, Ameredes BT, Bacharier L, et al. Characterization of the severe asthma phenotype by the National Heart, Lung, and Blood Institute's Severe Asthma Research Program. *J Allergy Clin Immunol.* 2007;119: 405-13.

10. Reddel HK, Taylor DR, Bateman ED, Boulet LP, Boushey HA, Busse WW, et al. An official American Thoracic Society/European Respiratory Society statement: asthma control and exacerbations: standardizing endpoints for clinical asthma trials and clinical practice. *Am J Respir Crit Care Med.* 2009;180:59-99.

11. Heaney LG, Conway E, Kelly C, Johnston BT, English C, Stevenson M, et al. Predictors of therapy resistant asthma: outcome of a systematic evaluation protocol. *Thorax.* 2003; 58:561-6.

12. Leggett JJ, Johnston BT, Mills M, Gamble J, Heaney LG. Prevalence of gastroesophageal reflux in difficult asthma: relationship to asthma outcome. *Chest.* 2005;127:1227-31.

13. Heaney LG, Conway E, Kelly C, Gamble J. Prevalence of psychiatric morbidity in a difficult asthma population: relationship to asthma outcome. *Respir Med.* 2005;99: 1152-9.

14. Busacker A, Newell JD Jr, Keefe T, Hoffman EA, Granroth JC, Castro M, et al. A multivariate analysis of risk factors for the air-trapping asthmatic phenotype as measured by quantitative CT analysis. *Chest.* 2009;135:48-56.

15. Sorkness RL, Bleecker ER, Busse WW, Calhoun WJ, Castro M, Chung KF, et al. Lung function in adults with stable but severe asthma: air trapping and incomplete reversal of obstruction with bronchodilation. *J Appl Physiol.* 2008;104:394-403.

16. Denning DW, O'Driscoll BR, Powell G, Chew F, Atherton GT, Vyas A, et al. Randomized controlled trial of oral antifungal treatment for severe asthma with fungal sensitization: The Fungal Asthma Sensitization Trial (FAST) study. *Am J Respir Crit Care Med.* 2009; 179:11-8.

17. Wenzel SE, Schwartz LB, Langmack EL, Halliday JL, Trudeau JB, Gibbs RL, et al. Evidence that severe asthma can be divided pathologically into two inflammatory subtypes with distinct physiologic and clinical characteristics. *Am J Respir Crit Care Med.* 1999;160:1001-8.

18. ten Brinke A, Ouwerkerk ME, Zwinderman AH, Spinhoven P, Bel EH. Psychopathology in patients with severe asthma is associated with increased health care utilization. *Am J Respir Crit Care Med.* 2001;163:1093-6.

19. Green RH, Brightling CE, McKenna S, Hargadon B, Parker D, Bradding P, et al. Asthma exacerbations and sputum eosinophil counts: a randomised controlled trial. *Lancet.* 2002;360:1715-21.

20. Haldar P, Pavord ID, Shaw DE, Berry MA, Thomas M, Brightling CE, et al. Cluster analysis and clinical asthma phenotypes. *Am J Respir Crit Care Med.* 2008;178:218-24.

21. Miranda C, Busacker A, Balzar S, Trudeau J, Wenzel SE. Distinguishing severe asthma phenotypes: role of age at onset and eosinophilic inflammation. *J Allergy Clin Immunol.* 2004;113:101-8.

22. Moore WC, Meyers DA, Wenzel SE, Teague WG, Li H, Li X, et al. Identification of asthma phenotypes using cluster analysis in the Severe Asthma Research Program. *Am J Respir Crit Care Med.* 2010;181:315-23.

23. Rackemann FM. A working classification of asthma. *Am J Med.* 1947;3:601-6.

24. Brozek JL, Bousquet J, Baena-Cagnani CE, Bonini S, Canonica GW, Casale TB, et al. Allergic Rhinitis and its Impact on Asthma (ARIA) guidelines: 2010 revision. *J Allergy Clin Immunol.* 2010;126:466-76.

25. Phelan PD, Robertson CF, Olinsky A. The Melbourne Asthma Study: 1964-1999. *J Allergy Clin Immunol.* 2002;109:189-94.

26. Limb SL, Brown KC, Wood RA, Wise RA, Eggleston PA, Tonascia J, et al. Adult asthma severity in individuals with a history of childhood asthma. *J Allergy Clin Immunol.* 2005;115:61-6.

27. Humbert M, Beasley R, Ayres J, Slavin R, Hébert J, Bousquet J, et al. Benefits of omalizumab as add-on therapy in patients with severe persistent asthma who are inadequately controlled despite best available therapy (GINA 2002 step 4 treatment): INNOVATE. *Allergy.* 2005;60:309-16.

28. Humbert M, Berger W, Rapatz G, Turk F. Add-on omalizumab improves day-to-day symptoms in inadequately controlled severe persistent allergic asthma. *Allergy.* 2008;63:592-6.

29. Wills-Karp M, Luyimbazi J, Xu X, Schofield B, Neben TY, Karp CL, et al. Interleukin-13: central mediator of allergic asthma. *Science.* 1998;282:2258-61.

30. Woodruff PG, Modrek B, Choy DF, Jia G, Abbas AR, Ellwanger A, et al. T-helper type 2-driven inflammation defines major subphenotypes of asthma. *Am J Respir Crit Care Med.* 2009;180:388-95.

31. Wenzel S, Wilbraham D, Fuller R, Getz EB, Longphre M. Effect of an interleukin-4 variant on late phase asthmatic response to allergen challenge in asthmatic patients: results of two phase 2a studies. *Lancet.* 2007;370:1422-31.

32. Slager RE, Hawkins GA, Ampleford EJ, Bowden A, Stevens LE, Morton MT, et al. IL-4 receptor alpha polymorphisms are predictors of a pharmacogenetic response to a novel IL-4/IL-13 antagonist. *J Allergy Clin Immunol.* 2010;126:875-8.

33. Wenzel SE, Balzar S, Ampleford E, Hawkins GA, Busse WW, Calhoun WJ, et al. IL4R alpha mutations are associated with asthma exacerbations and mast cell/IgE expression. *Am J Respir Crit Care Med.* 2007;175:570-6.

34. Corren J, Busse W, Meltzer EO, Mansfield L, Bensch G, Fahrenholz J, et al. A randomized, controlled, phase 2 study of AMG 317, an IL-4R alpha antagonist, in patients with asthma. *Am J Respir Crit Care Med.* 2010;181:788-96.

35. Hastie AT, Moore WC, Meyers DA, Vestal PL, Li H, Peters SP, et al. Analyses of asthma severity phenotypes and inflammatory proteins in subjects stratified by sputum granulocytes. *J Allergy Clin Immunol.* 2010;125:1028-36.

36. Lajoie S, Lewkowich IP, Suzuki Y, Clark JR, Sproles AA, Dienger K, et al. Complement-mediated regulation of the IL-17A axis is a central genetic determinant of the severity of experimental allergic asthma. *Nat Immunol.* 2010;11:928-35.

37. McKinley L, Alcorn JF, Peterson A, Dupont RB, Kapadia S, Logar A, et al. TH17 cells mediate steroid-resistant airway inflammation and airway hyperresponsiveness in mice. *J Immunol.* 2008;181:4089-97.

38. van Veen IH, Ten Brinke A, Gauw SA, Sterk PJ, Rabe KF, Bel EH. Consistency of sputum eosinophilia in difficult-to-treat asthma: a 5-year follow-up study. *J Allergy Clin Immunol.* 2009;124:615-7.

39. Cowburn AS, Sladek K, Soja J, Adamek L, Nizankowska E, Szczeklik A, et al. Over-expression of leukotriene C4 synthase in bronchial biopsies from patients with aspirin-intolerant asthma. *J Clin Invest.* 1998;101:834-46.

40. Sladek K, Dworski R, Soja J, Sheller JR, Nizankowska E, Oates JA, et al. Eicosanoids in bronchoalveolar lavage fluid of aspirin-intolerant patients with asthma after aspirin challenge. *Am J Respir Crit Care Med.* 1994;149:940-6.

41. Dahlén B, Nizankowska E, Szczeklik A, Zetterström O, Bochenek G, Kumlin M, et al. Benefits from adding the 5-lipoxygenase inhibitor zileuton to conventional therapy in aspirin-intolerant asthmatics. *Am J Respir Crit Care Med.* 1998;157:1187-94.

42. Dahlén SE, Malmström K, Nizankowska E, Dahlén B, Kuna P, Kowalski M, et al. Improvement of aspirin-intolerant asthma by montelukast, a leukotriene antagonist: a randomized, double-blind, placebo-controlled trial. *Am J Respir Crit Care Med.* 2002; 165:9-14.

43. Haldar P, Brightling CE, Hargadon B, Gupta S, Monteiro W, Sousa A, et al. Mepolizumab and exacerbations of refractory eosinophilic asthma. *N Engl J Med.* 2009;360:973-84.

44. Nair P, Pizzichini MM, Kjarsgaard M, Inman MD, Efthimiadis A, Pizzichini E, et al. Mepolizumab for prednisone-dependent asthma with sputum eosinophilia. *N Engl J Med.* 2009;360:985-93.

45. Simpson JL, Powell H, Boyle MJ, Scott RJ, Gibson PG. Clarithromycin targets neutrophilic airway inflammation in refractory asthma. *Am J Respir Crit Care Med.* 2008;177:148-55.

46. Simpson JL, Scott RJ, Boyle MJ, Gibson PG. Differential proteolytic enzyme activity in eosinophilic and neutrophilic asthma. *Am J Respir Crit Care Med.* 2005;172:559-65.

47. Baines KJ, Simpson JL, Bowden NA, Scott RJ, Gibson PG. Differential gene expression and cytokine production from neutrophils in asthma phenotypes. *Eur Respir J.* 2010; 35:522-31.

Economic Burden of Difficult Asthma

Ciaran O'Neill, Claire Telford

INTRODUCTION

Establishing the economic burden associated with a disease can be useful for a variety of reasons. Such information can help draw attention to a disease by highlighting the magnitude of the resources consumed, whether directly due to diagnosis and treatment or indirectly in terms of costs to society arising from productivity losses associated with morbidity and premature mortality. Quantifying the impact of a disease in monetary terms allows engagement of policy makers, using measures with which they are more familiar, and allows comparison with other diseases where similar data are available. The value of this should not be underestimated especially within a climate where competition for healthcare resources is increasingly fierce.

Beyond advocacy, a detailed characterization of the economic impact of a disease can provide insights into how healthcare systems confront it. Comparative analysis of resource use within a system can highlight inequities and may allow us to identify the impact of differential entitlements to care on the use of services, morbidity, and mortality. In addition, detailed understanding of where costs fall can also inform the development of evidence-based treatment assessment and diagnostic protocols.

A third rationale for the conduct of economic analyses is to identify where and how new technologies, including new drugs would fit into the current pathways for the diagnosis and treatment of a disease. While examination of the economic burden of a disease will not specifically address the cost-effectiveness of a new therapy, it may allow us to identify potential savings which might arise if a new therapy were to be introduced. This is particularly relevant in refractory asthma, where many of the potential new therapies are likely to be significantly more expensive than current treatments.

METHODS OF ASCERTAINING ECONOMIC BURDEN

Before examining the economic burden of difficult asthma, it is important to understand how costs are categorized in studies which examine economic burden, along with the usual methods used to quantify costs. This is useful to compare studies where cost estimates may differ because of the methods used rather than genuine differences in the economic burden of the disease.

In general, when considering the economic burden of a disease, it is the additional burden, i.e., additional to that expected for an otherwise healthy individual, which is of interest. Identification of this additional burden is undertaken in one of two ways, with the method used dependent on the type of data available. The methods are as follows:

1. Cost related to service utilization specifically due to the disease in question is collected and analyzed.
2. All service utilization by all individuals is collected and comparisons are then made between subjects with and without a specific disease and nonsufferers.

Costs are usually divided into two categories: those related to the diagnosis and care of the disease (sometimes referred to as direct costs) and those that relate to productivity losses that arise as a result of work time lost due to treatment, morbidity, or premature mortality associated with the disease (sometimes referred to as societal costs). The latter may also include work time lost as a result of the provision of informal care provided to children, e.g., a parent takes time off work to take care for a child who is absent from school.

While direct costs may fall largely on third party payers—namely the state or health insurer—significant elements may also fall on the patient in the form of out of pocket expenses related to co-payments, travel costs, over the counter medicines or complimentary therapies not covered by insurance plans or a publicly funded healthcare system. It is also worth noting that direct costs can relate to social or community services as well, depending on the healthcare system.

Where direct costs are established using a bottom-up approach—i.e., using individual patient level data—an approach known as activity-based costing is generally employed. Using this, activities that are associated with the diagnosis and treatment of a disease are identified, i.e., the care pathway is set out in terms of the activities that can happen along it. Next, the number of these activities, which individuals consume over a specified time period is measured. Measurements can be generated in a variety of ways including retrospective surveys of patients, review of patient charts, and use of administrative databases, e.g., those used for reimbursement purposes by third party payers. A tool which is popular in UK for collection of information on costs and service utilization is the Client Service Receipt Inventory,[1] in which information is collected retrospectively from the patient or the principal carer.

Each of the above methods of data capture has its limitations and cannot provide a complete picture of overall resource use. For example, while administrative databases (which have been widely used in this area) collect large scale data in a systematic fashion, they are unlikely to contain details of activities that generate out of pocket expenses for the individual. Similarly, while patient surveys may provide details on out of pocket expenses alongside patient-based estimates of activity covered by third party payers–hospital episodes, doctor office visits, or contacts etc., these may be less accurate than administrative databases, relying as they do on patient recall.

Once activity is measured, it is then monetized by the application of unit costs for each individual activity. These unit costs are usually obtained from reference costs produced for a particular jurisdiction. Where reference costs do not exist, the researcher may have to generate estimates of such costs, for example, through a survey of practitioners. This can be problematic, as unrepresentative practitioner samples, different knowledge base, and differences in terms of 'mark up' they apply to a particular service can produce variation. For example, it has been shown that teaching hospitals, operating as regional referral centres, incur higher overheads spread for pediatric asthma services.[2]

For direct costs incurred by the patient, a problematic issue may be recall bias on the part of the patient. While it can be managed to some extent by adjusting the time period that the survey question refers to, for example, 6 months for less frequent episodes of care, such as hospital stays or perhaps 4 weeks for more frequent episodes such as doctor office visits, the problem of recall bias will remain. If the service user is a child, who is particularly prone to asthma, it may be possible to have the principal carer provide the required information.

The same issue will apply to other costs where, for example, absences from work are identified by direct survey; however, additional practical and theoretical issues arise. In valuing absenteeism, an approach that is often used is to apply the earnings of the individual or average earnings (where issues may arise concerning reliability of reported earnings) in the jurisdiction for which the calculations are being made. This approach is grounded in what economists refer to as human capital theory, where the value of an individual's time is approximated by his/her earnings. Missing from this calculation is the cost of what is referred to as "presenteeism," that is, the productivity lost as a result of the individual being present but unable to perform his/her tasks as well as, would be the case in the absence of the disease. Because of the difficulties associated with making such estimates, costs related to presenteeism are generally not included in studies of economic burden.

For dependent minors, absences from school are often assumed to require absences from work on the part of the parent or guardian. Here again individual or average earnings (or some fraction of those) might be used to value lost productivity. However, two issues arise with this approach. Firstly, where absences from work are short or where the absence from work is longer but there exists less than full employment in the economy, using the human capital approach may overestimate the production lost as a result of work absences. In the case of short absences, it is possible, for example, that the absent individual's work can be covered on a temporary basis by existing staff. Similarly, where absence from work is of a longer duration, temporary staff may be employed from among those currently unemployed to cover the absence. In either case, the production lost as a result of the absence would be somewhat less than that suggested by their full earnings. This is why some researchers use a fraction cost approach to value lost production associated with sick days or lost school days. In this only a fraction of earnings are assumed to be lost.

The second issue concerns the valuation of time for individuals who are not economically active and whose episodes of illness does not involve absence from work (or absence from work of another to provide informal care). For a disease like asthma, many of those affected will be economically active and estimates of lost production may be substantial, whereas for other illnesses (for example, those that impact on older people, where informal care may not be needed or provided by another economically inactive person), estimates of lost production will be comparatively small. Because of the obvious equity issue, which would surround budgetary decisions based on these costs, and the fact that savings from these costs associated with the introduction of a new therapy are rarely reflected in health budgets, lost productivity does not attract the same attention as direct healthcare related costs in discussion of economic burden. Indeed, several jurisdictions (including the National Institute of Clinical Excellence in the UK) explicitly exclude such costs when considering the cost-effectiveness of new therapies. Such costs are nevertheless real and represent a significant component of the economic burden arsing from a disease.

Three final points are worth noting before considering the existing evidence on the economic burden of difficult asthma.

1. An important aspect of the economic burden of a disease is what is sometimes referred to as the intangible cost of illness—cost incurred by individuals in terms of impaired functioning or impaired health-related quality of life. Such costs are real in the sense that individuals typically place a positive value on health or in the case of chronic conditions, the alleviation of symptoms that attend poor health. By extension, the persistence of poor health has a negative value or cost associated with them. Such values, however, are not typically incorporated into estimates of economic burden in monetary terms, as it is difficult to apply a monetary value in a valid and consistent manner. In practice, therefore, it is usual for such aspects of disease burden to be expressed using measures, such as disability adjusted life years or quality adjusted life years. While it is recognized that such costs are real; indeed, it is reported that between 80 and 85% of asthma deaths occur in patients with poorly controlled severe disease,[3] these are not examined in what follows.

2. Estimates of the economic burden generally present a snapshot of costs at a particular time point and for a particular jurisdiction. They do not typically present the lifetime costs associated with treatment of a particular disease, which in the case of chronic conditions, such as asthma would typically be substantially more. While cost in a particular year may be a good reflection of those in subsequent or preceding years, this is conditional on technology, disease prevalence and access to care remaining stable. On a year-to-year basis, this may be a reasonable assumption, but the older the data are, the more tenuous the extrapolations based on it may be.

3. Related to the issue of disease outcome is that of adherence to medication and other treatment advice, which is very relevant to difficult asthma. Failure to take medication or take it in the manner prescribed, may not only result in poorer outcome but generate potentially avoidable costs elsewhere in the healthcare system, e.g., unscheduled doctor visits or hospitalizations. In difficult asthma, where a complex mix of therapies may be used, adherence may present a particular issue that may complicate comparisons across jurisdictions. For example, individuals in one jurisdiction may receive therapies fully funded through the public healthcare system, whereas in other jurisdictions these either involve a substantial co-payment or are only available if covered by private insurance or purchased 'out of pocket.' If all else is equal, the more directly the cost felt by the individual, the greater is the economic incentive to not comply/adhere with treatment. Differences in adherence, however, may contribute to differences in cost estimates across jurisdictions.

ECONOMIC BURDEN OF DIFFICULT ASTHMA

As with all economic analyses, it is important to try and understand the patient population, which is being studied and this is particularly relevant in difficult asthma. Some studies make the distinction between asthma severity and symptom control,[4] where asthma severity refers to the burden of symptoms in the absence of treatment, while control refers to the burden of symptoms in the presence of appropriate treatment. While the two are related, for example, maintaining control will likely become more difficult as severity increases, they are nevertheless distinct. Definitions of difficult or refractory asthma describe clinical situations where symptoms persist in the presence of high-dose therapy.[5,6] While these definitions try to be precise in terms of treatment, other definitions are used in the literature to characterize patient populations, including patient self-reported control,[7] a combination of patient reported control and objective symptoms measures, as well as use of specific healthcare resources.[8-10] In some studies, the patient population is more difficult to discern with precision.[11,12] This variation in terminology and patient population presents a major challenge when trying to compare studies and estimate of the economic burden of difficult asthma.

Other differences between studies are also evident, the relevance of which has been discussed at the beginning of this chapter, including:

- Different healthcare systems in which an individual study was conducted
- Different study year to which data relates (studies cited here span 1998[9] through to 2004[8])—this is a time period over which aspects of care may well have evolved
- Different age group of asthma patients in studies, e.g., Van Ganse et al.[9] limit the upper age of his subject group to 50, Lai et al.[7] and Sullivan et al.[8] allow for the inclusion of older patients
- Differences in recruitment strategy for patient data which might also impact on results.

Thus, as the authors need to control for so many factors, comparing the costs across individual studies that are subject to considerable heterogeneity is not always possible. The authors, therefore, restrict themselves to a within study comparison of the cost of uncontrolled and controlled asthma while reporting the magnitude of differences between studies.

COST OF UNCONTROLLED ASTHMA

Sullivan et al.[8] examined direct costs related to emergency room visits, inpatient stays, unscheduled physician visits, and asthma medications, as well as indirect costs related to absences from work due to illness or as a carer in the case of school days lost for a child. This study was conducted in the USA and costs were estimated on an annual basis over the course of two years.

Mean total costs for uncontrolled patients were over twice those of controlled patients in the 12 months following baseline assessment and in the second 12-month period, the difference exhibited a slight increase. For indirect costs, the difference was more marked. At 12 months, for example, the indirect costs of those with controlled disease were just over 6% of those with uncontrolled disease, while in the second year they were just over 2%.[8] For direct costs, a similar but less marked pattern emerged over time, with direct costs for uncontrolled patients rising for the second 12 month period. While it is dangerous to draw too many inferences with observations at just two time points beyond baseline, the observed pattern is consistent with a widening in the gap of the economic burden of asthma between controlled and uncontrolled asthma patients over time.

Within group analysis by these authors also revealed that as the level of poor control increased, so did the relative economic burden. For those with more than three markers of poor control (measured on the Adult Asthma Therapy Assessment Questionnaire), the burden of asthma increased from 2 to 3.5 times. As noted by the authors this again "...underscores the impact of control on patient outcomes and the cost of managing this disease...."

Van Ganse et al.[9] focused solely on direct costs in France, but produced similar findings in terms of the relative magnitude of poor control and relationship with the economic burden of asthma. Average direct costs over the course of 12 months for those assessed to have poorly controlled disease were 2.5 times that of patients whose disease was assessed to be well controlled. A pattern of higher costs among poorly controlled patients was evident across patients at varying levels of asthma severity, though interestingly the difference in costs was most marked among patients whose disease severity was assessed as being low (those with low severity and poor control had costs 3.5 times that of those with good control and low severity, while those with high severity and poor control had costs 2.9 times for that of those with high severity and good control).

Lai et al.[7] performed their analysis in China, Hong Kong, Korea, Malaysia, Philippines, Singapore, Taiwan, and Vietnam. Given the sampling approach used, it is difficult to be certain how representative the findings are for any of these countries. Both direct and indirect costs were examined though the indirect costs were confined to sick days, with no attempt apparently being made to calculate costs associated with informal care provided by parents. Average total costs among those who assessed their disease to be uncontrolled were more than 50% higher than those of respondents who considered their disease to be controlled; this difference remained when the authors controlled for a range of variables including severity and age. In this study, the difference in direct costs was more marked, with those with uncontrolled disease having average costs more than twice those of patients with controlled disease, though here there was no controlling for potentially confounding variables. Interestingly, while the average annual "maintenance" costs of these two groups were broadly comparable, there was an approximately threefold difference in "urgent" costs. As the terms "maintenance" and "urgent" are not clearly defined, some caution is warranted in the interpretation of these findings.

Other studies including those by Van Ganse et al.,[4] Piecoro et al.,[13] Antonicelli et al.,[11] and Stock et al.,[12] have all associated poor asthma control with higher costs. As the focus of these papers was not to identify the economic burden of difficult asthma, the authors generally did not identify the incremental burden attributable to poor control with increasing levels of therapy.

In the study by Van Ganse et al., the persistence of symptoms and utilization levels of inhaled corticosteroids to define severity was examined across three European countries, France, Italy, and Spain.[4] While poor control was evident and differences between countries identified, the impact of control on costs was not commented on specifically. However, it was asserted that poor control in patients with moderate and severe asthma correlated with higher costs among these groups relative to those classed as having intermittent or mild asthma. This provided indirect evidence at least of a relationsip between poor control and increasing cost. The study by Antonicelli et al.[11] used a subset of the data from Van Ganse et al.[4] (that for Italy) to examine the relationship between severity and costs. Not surprisingly, perhaps it reached similar conclusions "..inadequate control was associated with the level of (asthma) severity..." While these authors did not speculate on the level of savings that would occur with better control they commented "....given the strong association between symptom-based grade and costs, the savings potential accrued from improvement in asthma management may be considerable from a societal, patient, and payer perspective....."

Stock et al. examined the societal costs associated with disease severity in Germany using a combination of claims based data from insurers.[12] Interestingly, these authors used sickness benefit claims as part of their estimate of indirect costs associated with absenteeism, which was not a normal practice among economists. As with Van Ganse et al.[4] and Antonicelli et al.,[11] the costs of poor control were not identified separately but the authors speculated that better control could avoid costs associated with early retirement—a significant component of their overall cost estimate.

Piecoro et al. again used claims based data with the specific focus confined to direct costs.[13] The data used were for a selected group of patients (Medicaid patients in one state of the US) and use of inhaled short-acting β_2-agonists on a daily basis was taken as indicative of poor asthma control. As the authors conceded, they were unable to control for severity and based assessments of control (and adherence) on prescribing patterns which need not necessarily reflect usage. Among those whose asthma was not controlled, emergency room (ER) visits and inpatient hospitalizations were greater compared to those whose asthma was deemed to be controlled. While the difference in ER visits was not significant when age, gender, and ethnicity were controlled for, inpatient hospitalizations were approximately 50% higher.

Looking at these studies collectively, it seems clear that even while allowing for the differences in study design and context, there is a significant additional economic burden associated with poor control of asthma. The burden relates to both direct and indirect costs, and there is evidence consistent with the assertion that as the additional cost associated with poor control increases, the longer the exposure to poor control continues.

Recent work by O'Neill et al.[14] in the UK, looked specifically at a group of patients with difficult asthma and examined the economic impact of non-adherence. The authors examined healthcare utilization among patients whose asthma was difficult because they were non-adherent with prescribed inhaled long-acting β_2-agonist/ inhaled steroid combination therapy, compared to those with well characterized refractory asthma (by definition adherent with therapy). Costs examined were confined to direct healthcare costs measured from a publicly funded system perspective and included medicines, hospital admissions, ICU admissions, and other unscheduled healthcare visits associated with asthma care over the course of 12 months. The authors found that compared to a group of patients with refractory asthma, additional healthcare costs in non-adherent subjects due to hospitalization and unscheduled visits, were effectively offset by the reduction in costs associated with reduced medication utilization. While the cost of the adherent group's use of inhaled combination therapy was 2.5 times that of the non-adherent group, their use of hospital services was 40% lower and sufficient to outweigh higher combination therapy costs.

The difference in treatment costs is interesting, in that it identifies the potential savings associated with better control of asthma were adherence to be addressed. The authors estimated the avoidable costs would be between 24% and 40% of annual treatment costs, if non-adherence could be tackled in the non-adherent difficult asthma group. This figure, whilst substantial, may be an underestimate as it ignores the impact on absenteeism and health related quality of life, which as we have seen above, may be significant.

Intervention studies looking at the efficacy of asthma treatments in gaining asthma control have recognized the importance of examining the cost-effectiveness of such treatments. For example, within the Gaining Optimal Asthma Control (GOAL) study,[15] Briggs et al. found the use of salmeterol/fluticasone propionate improved control in asthmatic subjects, which resulted in QALY gains and reduced primary and secondary healthcare resource use (not including medications). Although patients from 44 countries entered into the study, unit costs were applied to the UK patients only and based on their analysis, the authors concluded that salmeterol/ fluticasone was cost-effective.

CONCLUSION

Asthma presents a significant burden in terms of its impact on health, health services, and the economy in the form of absenteeism. Evidence from a number of studies conducted in a variety of different settings, demonstrates that those whose asthma is poorly controlled contribute disproportionately to the economic burden of the disease, both in terms of healthcare resource use and lost productivity. While not all asthma may be amenable to control, several studies including those by Piecoro et al.,[13] Antonicelli et al.,[11] Van Ganse et al.,[4] and O'Neill et al.[14] indicate that adherence to treatment and/or treatment guidelines may be sub-optimal for a significant proportion of asthmatics including those with difficult-to-treat asthma. The corollary of this is that a significant proportion of the burden of difficult asthma may be avoidable.

As healthcare resources come under increasing pressure and as our understanding of the economic drivers in disease and the role of poor treatment adherence improves, so the issue of avoidable costs will come under increasing scrutiny. Why patients are non-adherent and how best non-adherence may be addressed are issues that warrant perhaps more attention than they have hitherto received by researchers and policy makers. While efforts should rightly be devoted to the development and delivery of new therapies, the potential of existing therapies may currently be unrealized because of a failure to address this issue. Confronted with a range of pressures that include population ageing, technological advance, and rising expectations, it is unlikely that even the wealthiest of our economies can continue to ignore this issue.

REFERENCES

1. Beecham J, Knapp M. Costing Psychiatric Interventions. In Thornicroft G, (ed). Measuring Mental Health Needs. 2nd ed., London: Gaskell; 2001. p. 200-24.
2. Meurer JR, Kuhn EM, George V, Yauck JS, Layde PM. Charges for childhood asthma by hospital characteristics. *Pediatrics.* 1998;102:E70.
3. Papiris S, Kotanidou A, Malagari K, Roussos C. Clinical review: severe asthma. *Crit Care.* 2002;6:30-44.
4. Van Ganse E, Antonicelli L, Zhang Q, Laforest L, Yin DD, Nocea G, et al. Asthma-related resource use and cost by GINA classification of severity in three European countries. *Respir Med.* 2006;100:140-7.
5. Chung KF, Godard P, Adelroth E, Ayres J, Barnes N, Barnes P, et al. Difficult/therapy-resistant asthma: the need for an integrated approach to define clinical phenotypes, evaluate risk factors, understand pathophysiology and find novel therapies. ERS Task Force on Difficult/Therapy-Resistant Asthma. European Respiratory Society. *Eur Respir J.* 1999;13:1198-208.
6. Proceedings of the ATS workshop on refractory asthma: current understanding, recommendations, and unanswered questions. American Thoracic Society. *Am J Respir Crit Care Med.* 2000;162:2341-51.
7. Lai CKW, Kim YY, Kuo SH, Spencer M, Williams AE. Cost of asthma in the Asia-Pacific region. *Eur Respir Rev.* 2006;15:10-6.
8. Sullivan SD, Rasouliyan L, Russo PA, Kamath T, Chipps BE; TENOR Study Group. Extent, patterns, and burden of uncontrolled disease in severe or difficult-to-treat asthma. *Allergy.* 2007;62:126-33.
9. Van Ganse E, Laforest L, Pietri G, Boissel JP, Gormand F, Ben-Joseph R, et al. Persistent asthma: disease control, resource utilisation and direct costs. *Eur Respir J.* 2002;20:260-7.
10. Peters SP, Ferguson G, Deniz Y, Reisner C. Uncontrolled asthma: a review of the prevalence, disease burden and options for treatment. *Respir Med.* 2006;100:1139-51.
11. Antonicelli L, Bucca C, Neri M, De Benedetto F, Sabbatani P, Bonifazi F, et al. Asthma severity and medical resource utilisation. *Eur Respir J.* 2004; 23:723-9.
12. Stock S, Redaelli M, Luengen M, Wendland G, Civello D, Lauterbach KW. Asthma: prevalence and cost of illness. *Eur Respir J.* 2005;25:47-53.
13. Piecoro LT, Potoski M, Talbert JC, Doherty DE. Asthma prevalence, cost, and adherence with expert guidelines on the utilization of health care services and costs in a state Medicaid population. *Health Serv Res.* 2001;36:357-71.
14. O'Neill C, Gamble J, Lindsay JT, Heaney LG. The Impact of Nonadherence to Inhaled Long-Acting β2-Adrenoceptor Agonist/Corticosteroid Combination Therapy on Healthcare Costs in Difficult-to-Control Asthma. *Pharmaceutical Medicine.* 2011;25:379-85.
15. Briggs AH, Bousquet J, Wallace MV, Busse WW, Clark TJ, Pedersen SE, et al. Cost-effectiveness of asthma control: an economic appraisal of the GOAL study. *Allergy.* 2006;61:531-6.

Clinical Assessment of Difficult Asthma

Annemarie Sykes, Andrew Menzies-Gow

INTRODUCTION

Difficult asthma comprises a heterogeneous group of patients who have persistent symptoms or frequent exacerbations despite being prescribed treatment at step 4 or 5 of the British Thoracic Society/Scottish Intercollegiate Guidelines Network (BTS/SIGN) management guidelines.[1] Clinical assessment of these patients can be challenging, as they encompass a number of clinical phenotypes, which have traditionally been poorly understood and frustrating to treat.[2-4] By the time patients with difficult asthma are referred to a specialist center, majority have been symptomatic for many years and subjected to multiple treatment trials with limited benefit, hence, the reason for referral. A systematic integrated approach to clinical assessment of difficult asthma patients is recommended[4,5] and the only way to untangle these complex patients.

The concept of systematic assessment was initially proposed in 1993;[6] however, formal guidance was not issued until the late 1990s when the European Respiratory Society (ERS) task force on severe asthma[5] and the American Thoracic Society (ATS) workshop on refractory asthma[4] suggested systematic assessment. The integrated approach recommended by the ERS task force included confirmation of asthma diagnosis, identification of the mechanism of persisting symptoms, and assessment of adherence to therapy. It was proposed that this system would enable difficult asthma specialists to better define clinical phenotypes, understand pathophysiology, and research novel therapies.[5]

SYSTEMATIC ASSESSMENT OF DIFFICULT ASTHMA

Systematic assessment is appropriate for all patients who have ongoing symptoms or lung function impairment at step 4 or 5 of the BTS/SIGN asthma guidelines.[1] There are several advantages of a systematic approach to the assessment of patients with difficult asthma. Patients are observed over a sustained period, usually several months, and a series of investigations performed, either as inpatient or outpatient, enabling the multidisciplinary team to monitor the patient when well and during periods of worsening disease control.

The patient's asthma diagnosis is tested and then confirmed or refuted. This allows identification of patients without asthma and rapid de-escalation of therapy and a search for alternative causes for their symptoms. Despite long-standing diagnoses and respiratory specialist care, a significant proportion of patients referred to difficult asthma services will not have severe asthma. Case series of referrals to services in London[7] and Belfast[8] found that 13[7] and 53%[8] of difficult asthma patients did not have treatment-resistant disease. Chronic obstructive pulmonary disease (COPD) was the most frequently identified alternative diagnosis and other conditions included cystic fibrosis, α1-antitrypsin deficiency, and cardiomyopathy.[7]

In patients with a confirmed severe asthma diagnosis, systematic assessment enables identification of any concurrent conditions that may contribute to loss of control or increased asthma severity. Comorbidities are common in difficult asthma patients; 34% of asthmatics in the Belfast case series[8] and 32% in the London case series[7] were reported to have coexisting disorders that produced asthma-like symptoms. Comorbidities identified in these studies are shown in table 3-1.

In confirmed asthmatics, the assessment process also involves evaluation of the patient's adherence to prescribed medications. Non-adherence with oral corticosteroid (CS) treatment, assessed by serum prednisolone and cortisol levels, is relatively common. In 36 difficult asthma patients, all prescribed at least 15 mg of prednisolone a day, 8 had undetectable serum prednisolone levels and normal

Table 3-1	Comorbidities Identified in Difficult Asthma Patients	
Comorbidity identified	*London[7] (% patients)*	*Belfast[8] (% patients)*
ENT pathology	51	95
Bronchiectasis	3	12
Psychiatric conditions	33	49
GERD	–	57
VCD	–	4
Dysfunctional breathing	–	9
Osteopenia	–	35
Osteoporosis	–	17
Pulmonary hypertension	1	–
Pulmonary eosinophilia	1	–
Extrinsic allergic alveolitis	1	–

ENT, ear, nose, and throat; GERD, gastroesophageal reflux disease; VCD, vocal cord dysfunction.

cortisol levels, suggesting prolonged non-adherence, with a further 6 having detectable prednisolone levels but normal cortisol levels, suggesting that these patients had only taken prednisolone on the day of blood test.[7] Detecting non-adherence is important to prevent further escalation of oral CS doses and the subsequent labeling of patients as steroid-resistant when the dose escalation fails to control symptoms. Confirmed asthmatics who are adherent to maximal medical management could potentially be candidates for steroid-sparing agents, anti-IgE, and other emerging targeted therapies.

Patients with difficult asthma are a complex heterogeneous group comprising several different phenotypes with differing clinical presentations, progression, and response to therapies. Systematic assessment facilitates better understanding of the different phenotypes and enables coordinated research, potentially leading to new therapeutic options and targeted treatment of different phenotypes.

The management of patients with difficult asthma is challenging and systematic assessment better equips clinicians to identify, characterize, and treat these patients.

SYSTEMATIC ASSESSMENT PROTOCOL

No agreed uniform protocol for assessment of difficult asthma exists, but it is recommended that evaluation should be performed through a dedicated multi-disciplinary difficult asthma service, by a team experienced in assessment and management of difficult asthma according to a protocol.[5] Figure 3-1 illustrates the potential outcomes of a patient referred for systematic assessment of difficult asthma and any protocol should focus on identification of these different groups. When complete, the results of history, examination, and investigations are discussed with the multidisciplinary team, when a clear diagnosis and management plan is made.

In the section below, the authors discuss the details of the clinical assessment protocol used at the Royal Brompton Hospital, London, UK.

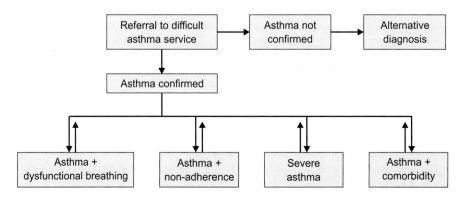

Figure 3-1 Potential outcomes of systematic assessment of patients with difficult asthma.

HISTORY AND EXAMINATION

Patients have usually been symptomatic for a prolonged period prior to presentation to a difficult asthma service and have often been reviewed by other healthcare providers who have been unable to fully control their symptoms. A clear logical history of their asthma is a vital part of the systematic assessment and the information received can alert clinicians to potential alternative diagnoses or comorbidities and also direct further investigation.

In addition to a standard medical history, a detailed account of the patient's asthma should be obtained, including age at onset, how the asthma diagnosis was established, and its progress since then. Pediatric and adult onset diseases are associated with different phenotypes; pediatric disease is predominantly atopic whereas, adult onset disease has a female and a non-atopic bias.[9] Adult onset disease, more common in patients with difficult asthma,[10] is a risk factor for chronic airflow obstruction[11] and has been associated with lower lung function and ongoing eosinophillic airway inflammations despite CS use.[12] Patients with late onset disease are also less likely to be atopic, have lower IgE levels, and fewer allergic symptoms.[13]

Regular peak expiratory flow (PEF) measurements over a sustained period of time and details of their best and worst PEF in the preceding year can indicate whether patients have chronic lung function impairment or have severe exacerbations with normal lung function inbetween.[14] Further indications of asthma severity and control are obtained from details of work absence, unscheduled physician visits, A&E visits, and hospital admissions due to asthma in the past year. Intensive care unit (ICU) admissions, including frequency and number of intubations, are also useful markers of exacerbation severity and, where possible, local ICUs are contacted regarding pressures required and tidal volumes needed for ventilation.

Details of a patient's known asthma triggers are sought, including nonspecific triggers, e.g., smoke, cold air, exercise, and infection, and other triggers, e.g., dust, pollen, foods, and animals, which suggest atopy. The relationship of asthma symptoms to menses, pregnancy, or menopause in females is important; although significant premenstrual worsening of symptoms is uncommon in difficult asthma patients,[15] it can be treated with hormonal manipulation.[16] Occupational asthma can also present as difficult asthma. Any relationship of asthma symptoms to the patient's occupations, present or past, should be sought, particularly improvement during weekends or holidays, as symptoms may be significantly improved by removing the patient from the work environment.[17]

Identification and treatment of comorbidities can potentially improve asthma control and their existence may be suggested by details in the patient's history. Allergy and atopy are less frequently identified in difficult asthma as opposed to milder disease.[10,18] Rhinosinusitis is common and chronic rhinitis, nasal polyposis, and sinusitis can all contribute to the severity of asthma symptoms.[19,20] Patients with difficult asthma also have increased sinonasal disease[20] and more sinus infections[10] than milder asthmatics and symptoms of perennial rhinitis are more common than seasonal symptoms.[10,18] Treating these may improve asthma control.[21]

Gastroesophageal reflux disease (GERD) is common in asthma[22] and patients with difficult asthma have increased GERD compared to milder asthmatics, with approximately 40% of difficult asthmatics reporting such symptoms.[10,15]

Obstructive sleep apnea (OSA) is also more common[19,23] in difficult asthma than in milder disease[23] and is associated with poor asthma control. Whether this relates to airway inflammation or obesity is unclear, but taking a sleep history and performing an Epworth sleepiness score can suggest OSA, which may contribute to nocturnal symptoms. In these patients, continuous positive airway pressure (CPAP) improves nocturnal symptoms[24] and quality of life.[25]

Details of past and present prescribed therapy are sought and whether medications were stopped due to side effects or treatment failure are identified. This is checked against what the patient actually took and for how long, potentially identifying inadequate treatment trials. Aspirin sensitivity suggests Samter's triad, which is associated with more severe asthma.[26] Anosmia and symptoms of nasal polyps also indicate increased severity of disease.[26] Systematic assessment also involves identification of steroid requirements, including usual maintenance dose and details of highest and lowest dose achieved, or frequency of oral courses in the last year.

Worsening of asthma symptoms can occur at times of major life events, so a detailed social history is also obtained, including recent stresses and those occurring at times of significant exacerbations. Smoking history, current and past, is obtained and smoking cessation is encouraged in smokers as, in addition to well described health effects, steroids appear less effective in smoking compared to non-smoking asthmatics.[27] Domestic animals can trigger asthma symptoms, and it is not uncommon for patients with difficult asthma to keep animals that they are sensitized to as pets.[7]

A full physical examination is performed as part of the systematic assessment of the difficult asthma patients. A thorough respiratory examination, including measurement of PEF and checking of PEF technique, can identify features that are consistent with a diagnosis of asthma, associated comorbidities, or alternative diagnoses. Crackles on auscultation can alert clinicians to bronchiectasis, pulmonary fibrosis, or heart failure. Widespread polyphonic wheeze is often present in asthmatics, whereas predominantly expiratory and upper airways noise suggests presence of an abnormal breathing pattern or vocal cord dysfunction. Clubbing does not occur in asthma and may indicate bronchiectasis, and a high body mass index (BMI) should raise the possibility of OSA.

Cardiovascular examination often identifies tachycardia secondary to inhaled β-agonists; however, the presence of raised jugular venous pressure (JVP), parasternal heave, peripheral edema, ascites, and hypotension can identify pulmonary hypertension as a comorbidity or alternative diagnosis. Eosinophilic lung disease can be associated with neuropathies and skin rash and a low-grade temperature can be evidence of chronic infection. Ear, nose, and throat (ENT) examination is performed in all patients, usually by an ENT specialist.

INVESTIGATIONS

Patients with difficult asthma undergo various targeted investigations. The choice of additional investigations is guided by information obtained from the history and examination. If consistent with an asthma diagnosis, the evaluation concentrates on adherence and identification of comorbidities; if not, the investigations concentrate on finding an alternative diagnosis. Table 3-2 illustrates potential investigations performed as part of systematic assessment of difficult asthma.

Table 3-2	Investigations Performed During Systematic Clinical Assessment of Difficult Asthma
Investigations performed	*Comment*
Blood tests	
Routine bloods, including CBC, U and E, LFTs, calcium, phosphate, and magnesium	General health status and presence of blood eosinophilia
Glucose and HbA1C	Detect steroid-induced diabetes
Immunoglobulins: IgG, IgA, IgM	Detect immune deficiency
Specific IgG levels to pneumovax and tetanus toxoid	Identify specific antibody deficiencies
Total and specific IgE: HDM, grass, cat, and others, as indicated from history	Identify potential allergic triggers
Aspergillus-IgE and -IgG	Indicate ABPA and chronic aspergillosis
ANCA and autoantibodies	Suggest Churg-Strauss syndrome and autoimmune conditions
ESR and CRP	Identify systemic inflammation
BNP	Possible heart failure or pulmonary hypertension
Serum prednisolone and cortisol levels (2 hr post dose), Theophylline levels (4–6 hr post dose)	Adherence to prescribed medications
Sputum	
MCS and AFB	Pulmonary infection
Eosinophil and neutrophil percentage	Support asthma diagnosis and indicate steroid responsiveness or presence of the neutrophilic phenotype

Continued

Continued

Investigations performed	Comment
Skin prick tests	
HDM (*Dermatophagoides ptereronyssinus*), grass pollen (*Phleum pratense*), Mugwort (*Artemesia vulgaris*), three trees, sliver birch, cat, dog, horse, *Aspergillus fumigatus*, *Cladasporium*, *Alternaria*	Identify atopy and potential allergic triggers
Radiology	
CXR	Identify alternative lung conditions
HRCT chest	
Pulmonary function tests	
Spirometry, lung volumes and gas transfer	Confirm diagnosis of asthma and assess current control. Identify other pulmonary conditions, including types I and II respiratory failure
Bronchodilator reversibility	
Histamine PC20	
Peak flow chart	
Arterial blood gas measurement	
Other investigations to consider	
Esophageal pH probe	Detect GERD
DEXA scan	Detect osteopenia/osteoporosis
Echocardiogram	Detect presence/severity of pulmonary hypertension
Overnight oximetry or sleep study	Identification of sleep disordered breathing
CT sinuses and ENT review	Detect sinusitis and polyps
Exhaled nitric oxide breath test	Indicate eosinophilic airway inflammation
Prednisolone absorption studies	Differentiate absorption problems from non-adherence
Bronchoscopy	Investigate alternative pathology, infections, and airway inflammation
Genetic testing	Detect cystic fibrosis
α1-antitrypsin testing	Detect α1-antitrypsin deficiency

CBC, complete blood count; U and E, urea and electrolytes; LFTs, liver function tests; HDM, house dust mite; Ig, immunoglobulin; HbA1C, glucosylated hemoglobin; ANCA, antineutrophilic cytoplasmic antibodies; ESR, enthrocyte sedimentation rate; CRP, C-reactive protein; MCS, multiple chemical sensitivity; AFB, acid-fast bacillus; BNP, B-type natriuretic peptide; ABPA, allergic bronchopulmonary aspergillosis; CXR, chest X-ray; PC20, histamine provocative concentration causing a 20% drop in forced expiratory volume in 1 second; HRCT, high resolution computed tomography; DEXA, dual-emission X-ray absorptiometry; GERD, gastroesophageal reflux disease; CT, computed tomography; ENT, ear, nose, and throat.

Sputum Examination

Sputum production is not universal in asthmatics and is associated with a more rapid decline in lung function.[28] Most productive asthmatics will describe clear mucous plugs. Dark, compressed, and powder like plugs can point to allergic bronchopulmonary aspergillosis (ABPA) and copious amounts of thick dark sputum can suggest coexistent bronchiectasis or cystic fibrosis.

Microscopy determines sputum cellularity, and culture can identify intercurrent infections. Detection of sputum eosinophils supports an asthma diagnosis and suggests a phenotype that may benefit from higher doses of oral CSs.[19,29] High eosinophils in sputum are associated with chronic airflow obstruction in older subjects with asthma,[12,19,30] and persistent sputum eosinophilia is a recognized feature of a subset of difficult asthmatics. A predominant sputum neutrophilia can suggest infective or occupational exposures.

Fractional exhaled nitric oxide (FeNO) is a marker of airway eosinophils; a nonlinear correlation exists between FeNO and sputum eosinophilia in severe asthma,[31] and levels are concordant with eosinophils on bronchial biopsies.[32,33] Despite this, the role of FeNO in difficult asthma remains undefined. Higher FeNO levels have been reported to be associated with lower forced expiratory volume in 1 second (FEV$_1$),[30] although other studies have not confirmed an association,[10,19] and several studies have found steroid treated patients with difficult asthma with the highest FeNO levels, suggesting that steroid therapy may be a confounder.[18,34]

Hematological Investigations

Blood tests are performed to identify comorbidities, assess adherence with prescribed therapy, and identify complications of treatment. The investigations commonly performed are described in table 3-2.

General health status and the presence of systemic inflammation can be indicated by complete blood count (CBC), urea and electrolytes (U and E), liver function tests (LFTs), and inflammatory markers (CRP and ESR). Low immunoglobulin levels or poor IgG responses to specific vaccinations can indicate immune deficiency associated with frequent infections or bronchiectasis. ABPA is suggested by raised IgE level and raised eosinophil count in association with positive *Aspergillus*-specific IgE and IgG. Autoantibodies and antineutrophilic cytoplasmic antibodies (ANCA) are performed to detect Churg-Strauss syndrome and other autoimmune conditions.

Blood eosinophil counts can be elevated in asthma. They drop quickly with oral CSs and are suppressed during treatment. A high eosinophil count in a patient prescribed oral CSs can indicate non-adherence. An alternative method of assessing adherence with CS treatment is by measuring serum prednisolone and cortisol levels. Adherent patients should have detectable prednisolone with reduced cortisol levels. Oral CS treatment has well recognized side effects and non-adherence with oral CS treatment is common in patients with difficult asthma.[7]

Pulmonary Function Tests

All pulmonary function tests are performed in patients with difficult asthma. Confirmation of the asthma diagnosis is a key component of systematic assessment and so in addition to lung function tests, bronchodilator reversibility and bronchial hyper-responsiveness testing is also performed. Spirometric measurements, pre- and post-bronchodilator administration, indicates level of pulmonary function and degree of reversibility. A reduced FEV_1, despite optimal treatment, is a common finding in severe asthma.[35] Bronchial hyper-responsiveness is assessed by bronchial challenge test, most frequently by inhaling double doses of nebulized bronchial irritants either histamine or metacholine. Although bronchospasm can be triggered in nonasthmatic individuals, severe asthmatics have pronounced airway hyper-responsiveness and a negative test should prompt investigations for an alternative diagnosis. Bronchodilator treatment prior to challenge testing can produce a false-negative result. Long-acting bronchodilators need to be withheld for 48 hours and short-acting bronchodilators for 24 hours prior to the test. Reversible airflow limitation and airway hyper-responsiveness is more marked in patients with difficult asthma compared to those with milder disease, but poor acute bronchodilator response has also been reported.[35]

In addition to lower FEV_1 and evidence of bronchial hyper-responsiveness, patients with difficult asthma have also been reported to have more obstructive spirometry, greater evidence of gas trapping, and mildly hypoxic and hypercapnic at rest.[18] Transfer factor is usually well preserved or marginally reduced, unless there is a significant prior smoking history.[15]

Imaging

All patients with difficult asthma undergo chest X-ray (CXR) and high resolution computed tomography (HRCT) scan to identify features consistent with asthma, such as air trapping and bronchial wall thickening,[30] and to indicate the presence of alternative or coexistent diagnoses. Bronchiectasis is the most frequently identified alternative diagnoses detected by imaging,[7] but other important comorbidities that can be suggested by HRCT include: ABPA, pulmonary hypertension, hypersensitivity pneumonitis, interstitial lung disease, and infections.

Skin Prick Tests

Atopy is less common in difficult asthma than in milder disease,[10] however, it is still present in more than 50% of patients.[15,18] All patients undergo skin prick testing to a panel of common aeroallergens (Table 3-2). Patients are commonly sensitized to house dust mite (HDM), grass pollen, and domestic animals[7] and specific IgE or radioallergosorbent tests (RASTs) can be performed to any potential triggers identified from the history.

Bone Densitometry

Long-term oral CS use is associated with osteopenia and osteoporosis, with one study reporting 34% of difficult asthma patients as osteopenic and 10% having evidence of osteoporosis.[15] Bone densitometry is performed on all patients to indicate the use of bone protective agents and potentially support the use of steroid-sparing agents.

Overnight Sleep Studies

OSA and sleep disordered breathing is common in difficult-to-treat asthma.[19,23] Many patients have raised BMI, exacerbated by long-term or frequent oral CS doses, which contributes to sleep apnea and impaired respiratory muscle function. Identification and treatment of associated sleep disordered breathing can improve nocturnal symptoms[24] and quality of life.[25]

Esophageal pH Monitoring

Approximately 40% of patients with difficult asthma report symptoms of GERD[10,15] and 30% have been prescribed a proton pump inhibitor (PPI).[15] Despite this, most will not have had an esophageal pH profile performed prior to referral to difficult asthma center.[15] Most patients undergo 24-hour esophageal pH probe to detect previously unidentified GERD or measure response to treatment. Treating GERD has been reported to have little overall effect on asthma;[36,37] however, treating patients with severe asthma with PPIs have shown some improvement on asthma control.[38,39]

MULTIDISCIPLINARY TEAM INVOLVEMENT IN THE SYSTEMATIC ASSESSMENT OF DIFFICULT ASTHMA

Systematic assessment of the difficult asthma patient involves clinical input from a number of healthcare professionals (Table 3-3).

Ear, Nose, and Throat Specialist

ENT symptoms are common in patients with difficult-to-treat asthma[8,10,15,18] and treating ENT symptoms may improve asthma control.[21] Chronic rhinitis, nasal polyposis, and sinusitis can all contribute to the severity of asthma symptoms.[19,20,26] Symptoms of perennial rhinitis,[10,18] sinus disease,[10,20] and previous ENT surgery[10,15] are more common in difficult asthma compared to those with milder disease. Review by an ENT specialist and examination by flexible fibroptic rhinolaryngoscope detects nasal pathology, such as cobblestoning of nasal turbinates, suggesting chronic rhinitis or thickening and inflammation of aryepiglottic folds, suggesting GERD, and allows direct visualization of the vocal cords enabling detection of vocal cord dysfunction (VCD).

Table 3-3	Multidisciplinary Team Involvement in the Assessment of Difficult Asthma
Member of MDT	*Assessment*
Asthma CNS	Assesses inhaler technique Discussion of asthma management plan
ENT team	Assesses contribution of upper airway to chest symptoms plus assessment for VCD
Respiratory physiotherapist	Assessment of breathing pattern at rest and during exercise, airway clearance technique education or review, and pulmonary rehabilitation
Health psychologist/ psychiatrist	Assessment of anxiety/depression and psychological contribution to symptoms
Dietician	Weight loss
Social worker	Social/benefits issues
Allergy specialist	Allergic contribution to symptoms
Smoking cessation clinic	Smoking cessation

MDT, multidisciplinary team involvement; CNS, clinical nurse specialist; ENT, ear, nose, and throat; VCD, vocal cord dysfuction.

Vocal Cord Dysfunction

VCD is the paradoxical adduction of vocal cords during inspiration, which results in intermittent extrathoracic airway obstruction and can produce attacks of severe dyspnea unresponsive to traditional asthma therapy. VCD was initially described as a 'non-organic' problem, predominantly affecting women with histories of abuse, that responded to speech and psychotherapy.[40] More recently, VCD has been recognized in elite athletes, military recruits, and children,[41] and there are reports linking VCD with GERD, laryngopharyngeal reflux (LPR), rhinitis, and post-nasal drip (PND).[41,42] The precise mechanism of VCD is unclear but current thinking suggest that irritants, such as chronic PND or reflux, leads to increased laryngeal sensitivity and hyperresponsiveness, and this causes accentuation of the glottis closure reflex and paradoxical adduction of the vocal cords in response to minor stimuli.[41] Symptoms of VCD can mimic those of asthma and is not an infrequent finding in patients with difficult asthma.[7,40]

The diagnosis of VCD can be difficult as patients' vocal cords can appear normal between attacks, can present with diverse symptoms difficult to distinguish from asthma, and patients can have coexistent VCD and asthma.[43] It is more common in females[44] and attacks usually occur suddenly, are self limiting, and of short duration. The history is often unhelpful although previous endotracheal intubation with normal inflation pressures raises the possibility of VCD.

Examination during an attack may identify inspiratory wheeze or stridor and lung function testing classically demonstrates inspiratory flow limitation or truncated flow volume loops. Metacholine challenge can provoke VCD and flattening of the inspiratory curve leads to reversal of normal midinspiratory flow (MIF_{50})/midexpiratory flow (MEF_{50}) ratio. A MIF_{50}/MEF_{50} of <1 is suggestive of VCD.

Lung function tests and flow volume loops can be normal, especially between episodes, so the current 'gold standard' for diagnosis is direct rhinolaryngoscopy. Inspection via a flexible fibroptic endoscope allows direct observation of paradoxical vocal cord movement, which can be accentuated by asking patients to perform a forced vital capacity maneuvre. Rhinolaryngoscopy also provides evidence of conditions associated with VCD, such as chronic rhinitis or GERD.

Management of VCD involves laryngeal relaxation and cough suppression exercises taught by respiratory physiotherapists or speech and language therapists and include techniques to abort VCD attacks. Identification and treatment of any associated conditions is also sensible. Treatment trials with heliox[45] or superior laryngeal blocks with *Clostridium botulinum* toxin[46] have been reported for patients with severe VCD.

Health Psychologist/Psychiatrist

A high prevalence of undiagnosed psychiatric morbidity has been identified in difficult-to-treat asthmatics[47] and psychological dysfunction is an independent risk factor for recurrence of asthma exacerbations.[19] Depression is particularly prevalent[47] and presence of depression, anxiety, external stresses, and secondary gain should be sought as part of the systematic assessment. In addition to patient's history, specific questionnaires can identify potential psychological problems. In 87 difficult asthmatics, the General Health Questionnaire (GHQ) identified 35 with potential for psychiatric problems.[7] Questionnaire-based assessments can have higher false-positive rates compared to psychiatric interview, but may be useful in excluding depressive illness.[47] Review by a psychiatrist or health psychologist is important for diagnosis and management of coexisting psychopathology. Psychoeducational interventions have been shown to have a small positive effect on hospital admissions in adults and there is limited evidence for an association between management of coexistent psychiatry morbidity and other asthma outcomes.[48,47]

Respiratory Physiotherapist

Assessments by respiratory physiotherapists can detect the presence of breathing pattern disorder and can educate sputum producing patients of the airway clearance techniques. Hyperventilation and other abnormal breathing patterns can coexist with asthma and result in symptoms out of proportion to the disease. Observation whilst talking or exercising can establish whether a patient's breathing is erratic, mainly nasal, or whether breathing involves predominantly upper chest wall movement. No formal studies have been reported till date on the impact of breathing control interventions in patients with difficult asthma.

Patients with productive cough can be taught airway clearance techniques and respiratory physiotherapists also liaise with local healthcare providers to organize pulmonary rehabilitation.

Asthma Clinical Nurse Specialist

The asthma clinical nurse specialist (CNS) has a key role in evaluation of the patients' understanding of their disease and in patient education. Inhaler technique is checked by direct observation and asthma plans and instructions are reinforced. Smoking cessation advice and support can be given where necessary.

SYSTEMATIC ASSESSMENT BY DIFFICULT ASTHMA SERVICES

The ERS task force recommends systematic assessment by a multidisciplinary team experienced in the investigation and management of difficult asthma patients; however, in practice, many difficult asthma patients are cared for by their local respiratory specialists. In an attempt to establish how difficult asthma patients outside specialist centers were cared for, a postal survey was sent to 683 consultant members of the BTS, requesting details regarding what resources were available to them and how they would manage four clinical scenarios.[49] Just over 50% replied and reported responsibility for 7,027 difficult asthma patients. Of the patients cared for by these specialists, only 20% had ENT review and 40% had a HRCT thorax. Only 25% routinely performed serum prednisolone and cortisol measurements and 14% did not perform skin prick test (SPT) to common aeroallergens.[49] Twenty-one of the respiratory consultants reported having a special interest in difficult asthma and 3,635 patients were cared for by these specialists.[49] Specialists cared for a mean of 173 patients each and were more likely to have access to SPT, psychiatry evalution, and prednisolone and cortisol assays than nonspecialists. Given these findings, it is logical that systematic assessment in a dedicated center with facilities for all the necessary multidisciplinary reviews and investigations is likely to be better for patients given their complexity, high symptom burden, and their large number of comorbidities.[7,10,15,18]

CONCLUSION

Investigation of difficult asthma can be challenging, but clear logical assessment of these patients can confirm the diagnosis, identify comorbidities, ensure best management, and assess adherence. More information is needed on the characteristics of different severe asthma phenotypes to guide future research in order to develop novel and more effective therapeutics.

Hopefully, within ten years, systematic assessment will be the cornerstone in planning targeted therapy for individual patients, to quickly improve disease control, minimize symptoms, and drug-induced side effects.

REFERENCES

1. BTS/Scottish Intercollegiate Guidelines Network. British Guideline on the Management of Asthma. *Thorax.* 2008;63:iv1-121.
2. Antonicelli L, Bucca C, Neri M, De Benedetto F, Sabbatani P, Bonifazi F, et al. Asthma severity and medical resource utilisation. *Eur Respir J.* 2004;23:723-9.
3. Serra-Batlles J, Plaza V, Morejón E, Comella A, Brugués J. Costs of asthma according to the degree of severity. *Eur Respir J.* 1998;12:1322-6.
4. Proceedings of the ATS workshop on refractory asthma: current understanding, recommendations, and unanswered questions. American Thoracic Society. *Am J Respir Crit Care Med.* 2000;162:2341-51.
5. Chung KF, Godard P, Adelroth E, Ayres J, Barnes N, Barnes P, et al. Difficult/therapy-resistant asthma: the need for an integrated approach to define clinical phenotypes, evaluate risk factors, understand pathophysiology and find novel therapies. ERS Task Force on Difficult/Therapy-Resistant Asthma. European Respiratory Society. *Eur Respir J.* 1999;13:1198-208.
6. Irwin RS, Curley FJ, French CL. Difficult-to-control asthma. Contributing factors and outcome of a systematic management protocol. *Chest.* 1993;103:1662-9.
7. Robinson DS, Campbell DA, Durham SR, Pfeffer J, Barnes PJ, Chung KF, et al. Systematic assessment of difficult-to-treat asthma. *Eur Respir J.* 2003;22:478-83.
8. Heaney LG, Conway E, Kelly C, Johnston BT, English C, Stevenson M, et al. Predictors of therapy resistant asthma: outcome of a systematic evaluation protocol. *Thorax.* 2003;58:561-6.
9. Bush A, Menzies-Gow A. Phenotypic differences between pediatric and adult asthma. *Proc Am Thorac Soc.* 2009;6:712-9.
10. Moore WC, Bleecker ER, Curran-Everett D, Erzurum SC, Ameredes BT, Bacharier L, et al. Characterization of the severe asthma phenotype by the National Heart, Lung, and Blood Institute's Severe Asthma Research Program. *J Allergy Clin Immunol.* 2007;119: 405-13.
11. ten Brinke A, Zwinderman AH, Sterk PJ, Rabe KF, Bel EH. Factors associated with persistent airflow limitation in severe asthma. *Am J Respir Crit Care Med.* 2001;164: 744-8.
12. Wenzel SE, Schwartz LB, Langmack EL, Halliday JL, Trudeau JB, Gibbs RL, et al. Evidence that severe asthma can be divided pathologically into two inflammatory subtypes with distinct physiologic and clinical characteristics. *Am J Respir Crit Care Med.* 1999;160:1001-8.
13. Miranda C, Busacker A, Balzar S, Trudeau J, Wenzel SE. Distinguishing severe asthma phenotypes: role of age at onset and eosinophilic inflammation. *J Allergy Clin Immunol.* 2004;113:101-8.
14. Ayres JG, Miles JF, Barnes PJ. Brittle asthma. *Thorax.* 1998;53:315-21.
15. Heaney LG, Brightling CE, Menzies-Gow A, Stevenson M, Niven RM; British Thoracic Society Difficult Asthma Network. Refractory asthma in the UK: cross-sectional findings from a UK multicentre registry. *Thorax.* 2010;65:787-94.
16. Redmond AM, James AW, Nolan SH, Self TH. Premenstrual asthma: emphasis on drug therapy options. *J Asthma.* 2004;41:687-93.

17. Vandenplas O, Dressel H, Wilken D, Jamart J, Heederik D, Maestrelli P, et al. Management of occupational asthma: cessation or reduction of exposure? A systematic review of available evidence. *Eur Respir J.* 2011;38:804-11.

18. The ENFUMOSA cross-sectional European multicentre study of the clinical phenotype of chronic severe asthma. European Network for Understanding Mechanisms of Severe Asthma. *Eur Respir J.* 2003;22:470-7.

19. ten Brinke A, Sterk PJ, Masclee AA, Spinhoven P, Schmidt JT, Zwinderman AH, et al. Risk factors of frequent exacerbations in difficult-to-treat asthma. *Eur Respir J.* 2005;26:812-8.

20. Bresciani M, Paradis L, Des Roches A, Vernhet H, Vachier I, Godard P, et al. Rhinosinusitis in severe asthma. *J Allergy Clin Immunol.* 2001;107:73-80.

21. Jani AL, Hamilos DL. Current thinking on the relationship between rhinosinusitis and asthma. *J Asthma.* 2005;42:1-7.

22. Gibson PG, Henry RL, Coughlan JL. Gastro-oesophageal reflux treatment for asthma in adults and children. *Cochrane Database Syst Rev.* 2003;(2):CD001496.

23. Julien JY, Martin JG, Ernst P, Olivenstein R, Hamid Q, Lemière C, et al. Prevalence of obstructive sleep apnea-hypopnea in severe versus moderate asthma. *J Allergy Clin Immunol.* 2009;124:371-6.

24. Ciftci TU, Ciftci B, Guven SF, Kokturk O, Turktas H. Effect of nasal continuous positive airway pressure in uncontrolled nocturnal asthmatic patients with obstructive sleep apnea syndrome. *Respir Med.* 2005; 99:529-34.

25. Lafond C, Sériès F, Lemière C. Impact of CPAP on asthmatic patients with obstructive sleep apnoea. *Eur Respir J.* 2007;29:307-11.

26. Ceylan E, Gencer M, San I. Nasal polyps and the severity of asthma. *Respirology.* 2007;12:272-6.

27. Tomlinson JE, McMahon AD, Chaudhuri R, Thompson JM, Wood SF, Thomson NC. Efficacy of low and high dose inhaled corticosteroid in smokers versus non-smokers with mild asthma. *Thorax.* 2005;60:282-7.

28. Lange P, Parner J, Vestbo J, Schnohr P, Jensen G. A 15-year follow-up study of ventilatory function in adults with asthma. *N Engl J Med.* 1998;339:1194-200.

29. Green RH, Brightling CE, McKenna S, Hargadon B, Parker D, Bradding P, et al. Asthma exacerbations and sputum eosinophil counts: a randomised controlled trial. *Lancet.* 2002;360:1715-21.

30. Bumbacea D, Campbell D, Nguyen L, Carr D, Barnes PJ, Robinson D, et al. Parameters associated with persistent airflow obstruction in chronic severe asthma. *Eur Respir J.* 2004;24:122-8.

31. Berry MA, Shaw DE, Green RH, Brightling CE, Wardlaw AJ, Pavord ID. The use of exhaled nitric oxide concentration to identify eosinophilic airway inflammation: an observational study in adults with asthma. *Clin Exp Allergy.* 2005;35:1175-9.

32. Payne DN, Adcock IM, Wilson NM, Oates T, Scallan M, Bush A. Relationship between exhaled nitric oxide and mucosal eosinophilic inflammation in children with difficult asthma, after treatment with oral prednisolone. *Am J Respir Crit Care Med.* 2001;164:1376-81.

33. Silkoff PE, Lent AM, Busacker AA, Katial RK, Balzar S, Strand M, et al. Exhaled nitric oxide identifies the persistent eosinophilic phenotype in severe refractory asthma. *J Allergy Clin Immunol.* 2005;116:1249-55.

34. Stirling RG, Kharitonov SA, Campbell D, Robinson DS, Durham SR, Chung KF, et al. Increase in exhaled nitric oxide levels in patients with difficult asthma and correlation with symptoms and disease severity despite treatment with oral and inhaled corticosteroids. Asthma and Allergy Group. *Thorax.* 1998;53:1030-4.

35. Chan MT, Leung DY, Szefler SJ, Spahn JD. Difficult-to-control asthma: clinical characteristics of steroid-insensitive asthma. *J Allergy Clin Immunol.* 1998;101:594-601.

36. Coughlan JL, Gibson PG, Henry RL. Medical treatment for reflux oesophagitis does not consistently improve asthma control: a systematic review. *Thorax.* 2001;56:198-204.

37. American Lung Association Asthma Clinical Research Centers, Mastronarde JG, Anthonisen NR, Castro M, Holbrook JT, Leone FT, et al. Efficacy of esomeprazole for treatment of poorly controlled asthma. *N Engl J Med.* 2009;360:1487-99.

38. Kiljander TO, Harding SM, Field SK, Stein MR, Nelson HS, Ekelund J, et al. Effects of esomeprazole 40 mg twice daily on asthma: a randomized placebo-controlled trial. *Am J Respir Crit Care Med.* 2006;173:1091-7.

39. Littner MR, Leung FW, Ballard ED 2nd, Huang B, Samra NK; Lansoprazole Asthma Study Group. Effects of 24 weeks of lansoprazole therapy on asthma symptoms, exacerbations, quality of life, and pulmonary function in adult asthmatic patients with acid reflux symptoms. *Chest.* 2005;128:1128-35.

40. Christopher KL, Wood RP 2nd, Eckert RC, Blager FB, Raney RA, Souhrada JF. Vocal-cord dysfunction presenting as asthma. *N Engl J Med.* 1983;308:1566-70.

41. Kenn K, Balkissoon R. Vocal cord dysfunction: what do we know? *Eur Respir J.* 2011;37:194-200.

42. Morrison M, Rammage L, Emami AJ. The irritable larynx syndrome. *J Voice.* 1999;13:447-55.

43. Parsons JP, Benninger C, Hawley MP, Philips G, Forrest LA, Mastronarde JG. Vocal cord dysfunction: beyond severe asthma. *Respir Med.* 2010;104:504-9.

44. Morris M, Allan P, Perkins P. Vocal cord dysfunction: Etiologies and treatment. *Clin Pulm Med.* 2006;12:73-86.

45. Reisner C, Borish L. Heliox therapy for acute vocal cord dysfunction. *Chest.* 1995;108:1477.

46. Maillard I, Schweizer V, Broccard A, Duscher A, Liaudet L, Schaller MD. Use of botulinum toxin type A to avoid tracheal intubation or tracheostomy in severe paradoxical vocal cord movement. *Chest.* 2000;118:874-7.

47. Heaney LG, Conway E, Kelly C, Gamble J. Prevalence of psychiatric morbidity in a difficult asthma population: relationship to asthma outcome. *Respir Med.* 2005;99:1152-9.

48. Smith JR, Mugford M, Holland R, Candy B, Noble MJ, Harrison BD, et al. A systematic review ro examine the impact of psycho-educational interventions on health outcomes and cost in adults and children with difficult asthma. *Health Technol Assess.* 2005;9:1-167.

49. Roberts NJ, Robinson DS, Partridge MR. How is difficult asthma managed? *Eur Respir J.* 2006;28:968-73.

4   Adherence in Difficult Asthma

Rob Horne, Liam G Heaney

INTRODUCTION

Asthma is a leading, preventable cause of morbidity, mortality, and cost, estimated to affect 300 million people worldwide.[1] Despite being prescribed treatment at Global Initiative for Asthma (GINA) steps 4 and 5, approximately 5–10% of adult patients remain difficult to control with persisting symptoms and frequent exacerbations.[2] There is increasing evidence that low adherence to maintenance treatment may be a significant contributory factor to difficult asthma.

Several recent UK studies have identified low adherence rates among patients referred to specialist centers for assessment of difficult asthma. In a Belfast study, 63 of 182 patients (35%) had filled <50% for inhaled combination therapy and 88% admitted low adherence after initial denial.[3] Low adherence was more common in females and associated with recurrent hospital admission and use of nebulized bronchodilators. In a Leicester study, 75 of 115 patients (65.2%) on inhaled corticosteroids (ICS) and 65 of 108 (60.1%) on inhaled long-acting β_2-agonists (LABA) had <80% prescription filling (Belfast study, <80% prescription filling was 64%).[4] Patients with low adherence had lower post-bronchodilator forced expiratory volume in 1 second (mean [SD] 75.4 [20.9] vs. 84.3 [23.5], p < 0.05), were more likely to have been ventilated for asthma (19.2% vs. 2.6%, p = 0.02), and had higher sputum eosinophils (geometric mean [log SD] 4.6 [0.66]% vs. 2.3 [0.54]%, p = 0.05). In a pediatric study from London, prescription filling was assessed as part of a home visit[5] with 30% of children filling prescriptions for <50% of inhaled maintenance therapy; medication issues encompassing adherence, an unsuitable device or poor technique were felt to contribute to poor control in 34 children (48%).

The situation is similar for oral steroid adherence. In the Belfast study, 25 of 51 patients (49%) were found to be non-adherent to prednisolone using a cortisol/prednisolone assay. Again, patients only admitted low adherence when "confronted" with objective measurements.[3] In another adult study, involving a London hospital in-patient assessment, 9 of 28 subjects (32%) prescribed ≥15 mg of prednisolone per day had either non-detectable prednisolone or non-suppression of cortisol.[6]

In the Leicester study, using prescription records alone, 13 of 50 (26%) had low adherence with oral prednisolone.[4]

It is important to note that many of these non-adherent difficult to control asthmatics are referred from other specialist physicians (Belfast study—37%, London Pediatric and Adult studies—100%), suggesting that this problem is not routinely identified during specialist assessment. These studies suggest that non-adherence in difficult asthma is not only as prevalent as in other long-term conditions but also a hidden problem. Moreover, in Belfast study, patients were initially reluctant to admit non-adherence until they were presented with precise prescription data. This has important implications for how low adherence is identified and managed in practice and these will be discussed later in this chapter.

IMPLICATIONS OF NON-ADHERENCE IN DIFFICULT ASTHMA

The first and most obvious consequence of significantly poor adherence is worse asthma outcome, particularly in terms of increased unscheduled healthcare use and increased near fatal events.[3-5] A further consequence of this is increased healthcare cost. Based on the Belfast data and assuming 5% of the 5.1 million UK asthmatics have difficult-to-control asthma, hospital admission reduction alone (including offsetting increased drug costs) could deliver a potential annual saving to the National Health Service (NHS) of *ca* £43 million annually.[7]

The next consequence of unidentified low adherence relates to our ability to identify and thus investigate therapy resistant or refractory asthma. Most definitions of therapy/resistant refractory asthma are based on failure to respond to high dose asthma therapy and thus predicated on adherence with this treatment,[2,8] but do not state how this should be assessed or addressed. The World Health Organization (WHO) statement on severe asthma acknowledged this problem and defined asthma severity on the basis of current clinical control and listed 3 situations where this could occur; untreated severe asthma (treatment not available, for example, due to economic reasons), difficult-to-treat severe asthma (the clinical problem where non-adherence, comorbidities, and other reasons may be the mechanism for persistent symptoms), and treatment-resistant severe asthma (where adherence has been demonstrated, hence "resistance" to currently available therapies).[9]

One consequence of an inappropriate diagnosis of "refractory" or "treatment resistant" asthma is that newer expensive therapies will be given to the wrong patient group. For example, the Health Technology Appraisal for Omalizumab from the National Institute of Clinical Excellence (NICE) stated that it should be given to subjects with severe persistent allergic asthma as an "add-on therapy to optimized standard therapy", with the latter described as "a full trial of, and documented compliance with, inhaled high-dose corticosteroids and LABA in addition to leukotriene receptor antagonists, theophyllines, oral corticosteroids and beta-2 agonist tablets, and smoking cessation where clinically appropriate" (http://guidance.nice.org.uk/TA133). Again, however, it is not stated how adherence should be assessed or identified.

In addition, to make omalizumab economically cost effective, NICE "targeted" the group of patients who were "expensive", specifically patients with 2 or more hospital admissions for asthma or 1 hospital admission plus 2 severe exacerbations requiring treatment/monitoring in an accident and emergency unit. Based on the Belfast study, where recurrent admission was more common with non-adherence, this stipulation potentially targets a non-adherent population. In this case, the most appropriate "treatment" would be to identify non-adherence and the reasons for non-adherence, and to attempt to support optimal adherence, rather than moving up the "prescription ladder" with more expensive treatments, which might also not be adhered to. The advent of novel expensive anti-eosinophilic therapies, e.g., mepolizumab could again theoretically "target" persistent airways eosinophilia in patients who are non-adherent with inhaled steroid therapy.

IMPROVING ADHERENCE: THE NEED FOR MORE EFFECTIVE INTERVENTIONS

Improving adherence is one of 10 priorities for reducing the burden of asthma on individuals and society identified in a recent European Union directive.[10] However, this seems to be easier said than done. A series of systematic Cochrane reviews have examined the efficacy of the most comprehensively tested adherence interventions across illnesses.[11] The good news that adherence can be improved is tempered by the bad news that even the best quality interventions do not seem to have major or sustained effects. For example, of 13 studies in asthma, only 6 reported improvements in adherence, and these were modest and short-lived.

A review commissioned by the UK National Institute for Health research augmented the Cochrane reviews by re-examining the papers and asking a different question: why have previous interventions had such limited effects?[12] This identified limitations in the way that previous interventions were developed and tested with important implications for the way forward. It concluded that although no single "off-the-shelf" intervention could be recommended, several principles could be applied to avoid mistakes and develop more effective solutions. The development of effective methods for supporting adherence has been hampered by misconceptions and myths about the reasons for non-adherence. Moreover, the size and scope of the literature on adherence can present a quite daunting prospect. The complexity of the topic is illustrated by the fact that there are 4 terms in common usage: compliance, adherence, concordance, and persistence (Box 4-1).

Box 4-1 Terminology—Compliance, Adherence, Concordance, and Persistence

Compliance is defined as the extent to which the patients' behavior matches the prescribers' recommendations. However, its use is declining, as it implies lack of patient involvement.

Adherence is defined as the extent to which the patient's behavior matches agreed recommendations from the prescribers. It has been adopted by many as an alternative to compliance, in an attempt to emphasize that the patient is free to decide whether to adhere to the doctor's recommendations and that failure to do so should not be a reason to blame the patient. Adherence develops the definition of compliance by emphasizing the need for agreement.

Concordance is a relatively recent term, predominantly used in the UK. Its definition has changed over time from one which focused on the consultation process, in which doctor and patient agree therapeutic decisions that incorporate their respective views to a wider concept, which stretches from prescribing communication to patient support in medicine taking. Concordance is sometimes used incorrectly as a synonym for adherence.

Persistence should not be confused with the term adherence. Persistence is the act of continuing a treatment for the prescribed duration and does not give an indication as to whether a patient adheres to the recommended timing, dose, or frequency. It may be defined as "the duration of time from initiation to discontinuation of therapy".

Source: Horne R. Compliance, adherence, and concordance: implications for asthma treatment. *Chest.* 2006;130:65S-72S.

UNDERSTANDING THE REASONS FOR NON-ADHERENCE: THE KEY TO EFFECTIVE INTERVENTIONS

Changing people's behavior is difficult. The Medical Research Council (MRC)[13] has developed guidelines for the development of interventions to effect behavior change in recognition of the difficulties and to help address the limitations of previous interventions. Central to the MRC recommendations is that intervention development is informed by an appropriate theory of behavior and behavior change.

Dispelling Myths

Virtually, none of the interventions to support adherence, included in recent Cochrane reviews have utilized specific theories of medication non-adherence. Indeed, many previous attempts to address the problem of non-adherence appear to have been based on myths about a framework for non-adherence to which we refer. To help understand why previous interventions have had limited effects and how we might improve future interventions, first we need to dispel some of these common myths about the reasons for non-adherence.

Myth 1: Non-adherence does not occur in severe disease. Non-adherence is not significantly related to the type or severity of the disease with rates of 25–30% noted across 17 studies.[14] Non-adherence rates of over 20% have been documented in potentially life-threatening conditions, such as cancer and HIV/AIDS.

Myth 2: The noncompliant patient. There are no clear, consistent links between non-adherence and sociodemographic variables in adults across illnesses.[15] Adherence is positively correlated with income when the patient is paying for treatment[16-18] but not with general socioeconomic status.[14] In fact, adherence rates vary, not just between individuals, but within the same individual, over time, and across treatments. Adherence is a variable behavior rather than a trait characteristic: we are all non-adherent some of the time. Even if stable associations existed between sociodemographic or trait characteristics, they would serve to identify certain "at risk" groups so that interventions could be targeted, but could do little to inform the type or content of these interventions. The challenge is to identify causes of non-adherence, which can be modified rather than fixed characteristics that cannot.

Myth 3: "Once a day" treatments solve the problem. Simplifying the regimen can certainly aid adherence, particularly if the regimen is complex or difficult to administer. However, non-adherence also occurs with once-a-day treatments. Although finding the most convenient and easy to administer formulation is an important aspect, this does not guarantee adherence. We need to look beyond formulation to how the regimen fits with the patients' lifestyle preferences and abilities.[19]

Myth 4: Providing clear instructions and improving knowledge will guarantee adherence. Providing clear instructions and improving knowledge, although essential is not enough to guarantee adherence. Often, in medicine, we tell patients what we want them to hear. This can create an information-action gap. People does not blindly follow health advice, even if it comes from trusted clinicians. Rather, we evaluate the advice and make a "commonsense" decision about whether to follow it. This will be covered in more detail later, but here it is sufficient to note 3 things:

1. In order to change behavior, information has to either concur with our beliefs about the behavior or change those beliefs: information needs to persuade as well as inform.[20]
2. Many patients are dissatisfied with the type and amount of medicines information they receive.[21-25]
3. Information should be targeted to the needs of the individual both in terms of content (what it says) and complexity, so that it addresses outstanding questions and conveys recommendations. It should match patients' own level of health literacy; their ability to obtain, process, and understand basic health information needed to make appropriate health decisions.[26]

A PERCEPTIONS AND PRACTICALITIES APPROACH

The perceptions and practicalities approach (PPA) provides a framework for moving beyond the myths of non-adherence to developing effective, patient-centered solutions (Figure 4-1). Its central tenets are:

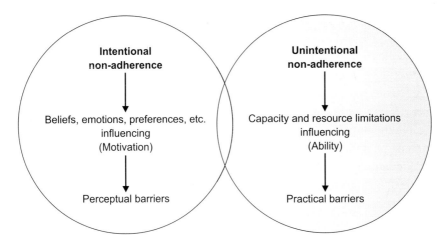

Figure 4-1 A perceptions and practicalities approach explaining non-adherence. *From* Horne R. Compliance, adherence and concordance. In: Taylor K, Harding G, editors. Pharmacy Practice. London: Taylor and Francis; 2001. p. 165-84.

1. The many causes of non-adherence fall into 2 overlapping categories: intentional and unintentional.

2. Unintentional non-adherence occurs when the patient wants to take the medicine but is prevented from doing so by barriers beyond their control, such as poor recall or comprehension of instructions, difficulties in administering the treatment, simply forgetting, or because they cannot afford it. Deliberate or intentional non-adherence arises when the patient decides not to follow the treatment recommendations. One of the few studies to explore the proportion of intentional vs. unintentional non-adherence found that in sample of UK patients, receiving a new medicine form a community pharmacy, over 44% of the reported non-adherence after 4 weeks was intentional.[27]

3. Unintentional non-adherence results from limitations in capacity and resources that reduce the person's ability to adhere. These are *practical* barriers. Intentional non-adherence can be understood in terms of the beliefs and preferences influencing our motivation to start and continue with treatment. These are *perceptual* barriers

4. To understand non-adherence and facilitate adherence, we need to consider both motivation and ability (resources). There is a degree of overlap between intentional and unintentional non-adherence. Motivation may overcome resource barriers and resource barriers may reduce motivation.

5. Each individual may have a unique mix of perceptual and practical barriers to adherence and interventions should be tailored to meet the needs of individuals by first assessing the specific barriers and then selecting appropriate techniques to address each barrier.

6. Perceptual and practical barriers require different types of interventions. For example, perceptual barriers might be addressed by cognitive behavioral techniques or motivational interviewing, whereas practical barriers might be overcome by interventions that increase capacity or improve ability (e.g., reminder systems to reduce forgetting).

7. The perceptual and practical barriers for each individual will be affected by sociodemographic, cultural and economic factors, and trait characteristics, such as personality.[28] However, the effect of these variables will vary among individuals. For this reason, the assessment of the specific perceptual and practical barriers for each individual should be the starting point for adherence interventions.[29,30] One size does not fit all!

PATIENTS' BELIEFS ABOUT MEDICINES: NECESSITY AND CONCERNS

Patients motivation to start and continue with prescribed medication is influenced by the way in which they judge their personal need for medication (necessity beliefs), relative to their concerns about potential adverse effects.[31,32] Necessity beliefs and concerns can be assessed using the Beliefs about Medicines Questionnaire (BMQ).[33] This brief questionnaire is valid and reliable across a range of long-term conditions, including asthma and can be completed by most patients in about 5–10 minutes. The BMQ has been used to assess patient perceptions of maintenance treatment in several studies involving patients with asthma,[32,34,35] and in each study, non-adherence was related to doubts about personal need for the treatment and concerns about potential adverse effects. Although we cannot extrapolate the findings from these samples of predominantly community-managed asthma patients into a difficult asthma population, they illustrate how patients' implicit evaluations of their maintenance treatment seem to influence adherence. The effect on adherence may be implicit as well as explicit.[36] For example, in some situations, non-adherence could be the result of a deliberate strategy to minimize harm by taking less medication. Alternatively, it might simply be a reflection of the fact that patients who do not perceive their medication to be important are more likely to forget to take it.

For example, in a sample of 3,916 patients with asthma recruited from 85 UK general practices,[37] there was considerable variation in patients' perceptions of about their personal need for ICS and about one-third were concerned about potential adverse effects (manuscript in preparation). One obvious source of concern is the experience of symptoms as medication "side effects" and the disruptive effects of medication on daily living, but this is not the whole picture. In the sample of UK community-treated asthma patients surveyed by Clatworthy et al.,[37] many patients who did not report ICS "side effects" were still concerned about possible problems in the future. Often, concerns were based on beliefs about the dangers of medication, including worries about long-term effects (44%), the risks of becoming too dependent on medicines (34%), and belief that ICS would become less effective in future if used regularly as prescribed (23%).

Necessity beliefs and concerns are salient perceptual barriers that could be addressed by interventions to facilitate uptake and persistence with ICS: prescribers need to counter doubts about personal need and address treatment concerns. However, to do this requires insight into the origins of these beliefs.

THE COMMONSENSE ORIGINS OF PATIENTS' BELIEFS ABOUT THEIR PERSONAL NEED FOR INHALED CORTICOSTEROIDS

In order to be convinced of a personal need for ongoing medication, we must first perceive a good fit between the *problem* (the illness or condition) and the *solution* (the medication). Patients' commonsense perceptions of illness influence their beliefs about the necessity of medication.[36] Most people do not blindly follow treatment recommendations, even when they are made by trusted clinicians. Instead, we tend to evaluate whether the advice makes "commonsense" in the light of their personal understanding and beliefs about the illness.[38] Although patients' commonsense models of illness may differ from the medical view, they have an internal logic and coherence, and influence illness-related behavior.[39]

Symptoms perceptions relative to expectations are important. Until we experience a chronic condition, most of our experience of illness is symptomatic and acute. We know we are ill because we experience symptoms. We know when we are better, because the symptoms go away. We carry these expectations of symptoms and illness with us when we encounter long-term conditions. For many long-term conditions, including asthma, the medical rationale for maintenance treatment is based on a prophylaxis model. The benefits of treatment are often silent and long-term. This may be in stark contrast to our intuitive commonsense model of "no symptoms no problem".[40] The importance of illness representation in adherence to ICS is illustrated by studies in the UK[32] and USA.[40] Many patients considered themselves to be well when asthma symptoms were absent and took ICS sporadically in response to symptoms. They doubted their personal need for preventer medication, because the notion of asthma as a *chronic* condition, needing continuous treatment, was at odds with their experience of it as an *episodic* problem. Moreover, missing doses did not lead to an immediate deterioration in symptoms, so reinforcing the (potentially erroneous) perception that high adherence to the medication may not be necessary.

Suspicion of Pharmaceuticals and Concerns about Inhaled Corticosteroids

ICS concerns are related to prototypic "background beliefs" about the nature of pharmaceuticals as a class of treatments.[33] Many people are suspicious of pharmaceuticals and the pharmaceutical industry. They tend to view all medicines as having common properties. The benefits of medicines are often taken for granted with a focus on the potential negative effects. In this view, medicines are often seen as intrinsically harmful addictive substances that are overused by doctors and the healthcare system. These "social representations" of medicines are linked to wider concerns about scientific medicine, lack of trust in doctors, and an increasing interest in alternative or complementary healthcare.[41]

General medication beliefs influence the way in which people evaluate *specific* medication prescribed for a particular medical condition (Figure 4-2).[42] They frame initial expectations of the outcome of taking the prescribed medication[43] as well as how subsequent events are interpreted—for example, whether symptoms are attributed to the illness or the treatment.[44] General beliefs about medicines may also contribute to perception of medication necessity and could even influence outcome directly through the placebo/effect although this has yet to be empirically tested.

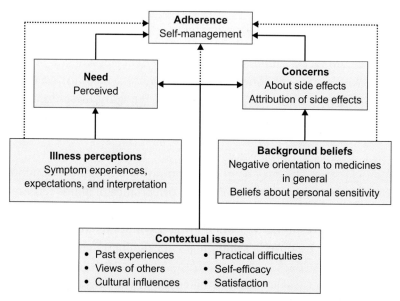

Figure 4-2 Patient adherence to medication is influenced by a number of factors relating to how the individual judges the necessity of their treatment relative to their concern. *From* Horne R. Compliance, adherence, and concordance: implications for asthma treatment. *Chest.* 2006;130:65S-72S.

MEMORY AND FORGETTING

Forgetting is the most commonly reported reason for treatment of non-adherence,[45,46] although this may in part be due to a reporting bias, as it may be more socially acceptable to disclose unintentional than intentional non-adherence. There are 2 separate memory processes linked to adherence—remembering the treatment instructions (retrospective memory) and remembering to take/engage in the treatment at the right time. Memory performance has been associated with adherence to medication across a range of chronic conditions, including HIV,[47] diabetes,[48] and chronic obstructive pulmonary disease.[49] Interventions using reminder systems to combat forgetting can be effective, but the effects are typically modest,[50,51] perhaps, because they fail to address perceptual barriers.

Other interventions designed to reduce forgetting, focus on the development of plans known as "implementation intentions."[52] Implementation intentions tie a specific adherence behavior to an environmental cue by planning how and when the behavior can be carried out. Turning an intention (e.g., "I will take my medicine") into a more specific implementation intention (e.g., "I will take my medicine every morning immediately after I clean my teeth"). This approach has been successfully applied to improving adherence to antiepileptic medication[53] but has yet to be used in difficult asthma.

OTHER FACTORS AND CHALLENGES

Emotion and affect are likely to influence both perceptual and practical barriers to adherence as well as individual responses to efforts to overcome them. A meta-analysis of 25 studies found that the relationship between depression and non-adherence to medication prescribed for chronic illnesses (other than depression) was substantial. Anxiety had little effect.[54] A further area for future research is the effect of social support. Social support appears to have broadly positive effects on adherence but we know little about the mechanism or the type of support that works best in what situations.

IMPLICATIONS FOR PRACTICE

The PPA to non-adherence has informed NICE medicines adherence guidelines,[55] developed to help health professionals support patients in making informed choices about and adhering to prescribed medication. The principle is to identify the specific perceptual and practical barriers to adherence for each individual and apply specific interventions to address the unique mix of perceptual and/or practical barriers for each patient.

This can be summarized in 3 steps:

1. Communicate a "commonsense" rationale for why the treatment is needed. Patients need to perceive a close fit between the problem (the illness) and the proposed solution (e.g., regular use of maintenance treatment), and to provide

a convincing "story" for why medication is still necessary, even when symptoms are not present or when symptom resolution is delayed.

2. Elicit and address patient concerns about the medication, help the patient make treatment choices that are informed by an understanding of the likely risks and benefits, rather than by potentially erroneous beliefs or misconceptions about the condition and treatment. It is important to understand this from the patients' perspective. For example, the patient may be worried about subjective side effects that clinicians may perceive to be clinically insignificant.

3. Identify and address potential practical barriers and to make the regimen as convenient and easy to take as possible.

Adherence support should occur, not just at the start of treatment, but also during treatment review as perceptions, abilities, and adherence can change over time. This requires a team approach involving clinicians, nurses, and pharmacists who can contribute through medication counseling and review.[56]

Adherence support should be "menu-driven", i.e., tailored to the needs of the individual. Using an approach in a small randomized controlled pilot study has recently shown that in 35% of patients referred to a tertiary center with low adherence as the primary cause of difficult to control asthma, identifying and "confronting" the problem in a medical concordance interview induced sustained behavioral change.[57] In those subjects with "persistent" non-adherence, a more complex menu-driven behavioral intervention also demonstrated improved prescription filling and a trend to better outcome. Such approaches need to be studied in multi-centered clinical trials, because if even moderately successful, they are likely to deliver a substantial improvement in outcome in this patient group.

IDENTIFYING NON-ADHERENCE: THE NEED FOR A "NO-BLAME" APPROACH

The first step remains the identification of non-adherence. Non-adherence is often a hidden problem; as the experience in Belfast shows, patients are often reluctant to reveal non-adherence and the associated doubts and concerns about treatment to clinicians for fear of offending them. Many patients believe that lack of faith in the treatment will be interpreted by the clinician as a lack of faith in the prescriber. It is important, therefore, to take a "no-blame" approach that facilitates honest disclosure of non-adherence and encourages patients to express doubts and concerns. The cheapest and easiest method is to ask patients; however, self-report is notoriously unreliable and inaccurate. However, the accuracy and reliability of self-report can be improved by communicating a "no-blame" approach that sanctions non-adherence.[32]

The Medication Adherence Report Scale applies this approach to elicit reports of non-adherence and low adherence identified with this scale has been shown to relate to poor asthma control[37] and electronic adherence measurement.[58]

However, as the Belfast experience shows,[3] patients may be unwilling or unable to acknowledge non-adherence unless they are presented with objective data. For such patients, feedback of actual adherence patterns may be a helpful intervention, if accompanied by a no-blame approach with concordance discussion and tailored support.[59] To this end, the development of biomarkers and/or objective tests of steroid exposure would be valuable in difficult asthma, where complex and expensive treatments are being considered. In terms of a potential biomarker, there are a number of genes which are rapidly and consistently upregulated after steroid exposure,[60] and some of these provide attractive targets to develop a marker of adherence to steroid therapy. It seems probable that any such biomarker, as with other objective measures of drug adherence, such as theophylline and prednisolone serum levels or the use of "smart inhalers", will have to be combined with other measures, such as effective self-report methods, surrogates, such as prescription filling, and coupled with a no-blame approach to discussion.

For clinical practice, the key challenge is to utilize these different measures to bring non-adherence out into the open by facilitating an honest and open discussion. Developing technological approaches, such as better detection methods, may facilitate this discussion, but is unlikely to deliver better clinical outcomes without better methods for negotiating treatments with patients and supporting informed choice and optimal adherence. Whilst low adherence is described as a potential mechanism for difficult-to-control asthma in national and international asthma guidelines, precise guidance on how this should be identified and managed has so far been absent.[61,62]

CONCLUSION

Non-adherence remains a significant problem in difficult-to-control asthma. There has been a failure to systematically implement processes and clinical tools, which have been shown to help identify and address non-adherence. The key challenge is to empower patients to make informed choices about medicines, rather than decisions influenced by misplaced beliefs about benefit and harm. There are many consequences of this failure but given the advent of novel expensive parenteral therapies for more difficult-to-manage asthma, it has now become imperative that non-adherence is targeted and clinical trials supported to examine interventions to address the problem in subjects with difficult asthma.

REFERENCES

1. Masoli M, Fabian D, Holt S, Beasley R. Global burden of asthma. 2003. Available from: http://www.ginasthma.com.
2. Proceedings of the ATS workshop on refractory asthma: current understanding, recommendations, and unanswered questions. American Thoracic Society. *Am J Respir Crit Care Medi.* 2000;162:2341-51.

3. Gamble J, Stevenson M, McClean E, Heaney LG. The prevalence of non-adherence in difficult asthma. *Am J Respir Crit Care Med.* 2009;180:817-22.

4. Murphy AC, Proeschel A, Linnett ME, Brightling CE, Wardlaw AJ, Pavord ID, et al. P174 Identifying non-adherence with asthma medication and the relationship to clinical outcomes amongst adults with difficult-to-control asthma. *Thorax.* 2010;65:A151.

5. Bracken M, Fleming L, Hall P, Van Stiphout N, Bossley C, Biggart E, et al. The importance of nurse-led home visits in the assessment of children with problematic asthma. *Arch Dis Child.* 2009;94:780-4.

6. Robinson DS, Campbell DA, Durham SR, Pfeffer J, Barnes PJ, Chung KF, et al. Systematic assessment of difficult-to-treat asthma. *Eur Resp J.* 2003;22:478-83.

7. O'Neill C, Gamble J, Lindsay JT, Heaney LG. The impact of nonadherence to inhaled long-acting β2-adrenoceptor agonist/corticosteroid combination therapy on healthcare costs in difficult-to-control asthma. *Pharmaceutical Medicine.* 2011;25:379-85.

8. Barnes PJ, Woolcock AJ. Difficult asthma. *Eur Respir J.* 1998;12:1209-18.

9. Bousquet J, Mantzouranis E, Cruz AA, Ait-Khaled N, Baena-Cagnani CE, Bleecker ER, et al. Uniform definition of asthma severity, control, and exacerbations: document presented for the World Health Organization Consultation on Severe Asthma. *J Allergy Clin Immunol.* 2010;126:926-38.

10. Holgate S, Bisgaard H, Bjermer L, Haahtela T, Haughney J, Horne R, et al. The Brussels Declaration: the need for change in asthma management. *Eur Respir J.* 2008;32:1433-42.

11. Haynes RB, Yao X, Degani A, Kripalani S, Garg AX, McDonald HP. Interventions for enhancing medication adherence. *Cochrane Database Syst Rev.* 2005;CD000011.

12. Horne R, Kellar I. Interventions to facilitate adherence. In: Horne R, Weinman J, Barber N, Elliott RA, Morgan M, editors. Concordance, adherence and compliance in medicine taking: a conceptual map and research priorities. London: National Institute for Health Research (NIHR) Service Delivery and Organisation (SDO) Programme. 2005 Available from: http://www.sdo.nihr.ac.uk/files/project/SDO_FR_08-1412-076_V01.pdf.

13. Craig P, Dieppe P, Macintyre S, Michie S, Nazareth I, Petticrew M. Developing and evaluating complex interventions: the new Medical Research Council guidance. *BMJ.* 2008;337:a1655.

14. DiMatteo MR. Variations in patients' adherence to medical recommendations: a quantitative review of 50 years of research. *Med Care.* 2004;42:200-9.

15. Horne R, Weinman J, Barber N, Elliott RA, Morgan M. Concordance, adherence and compliance in medicine taking: a conceptual map and research priorities. 2006. Available from: http://www.sdo.lshtm.ac.uk/files/project/76-final-report.pdf.

16. Hirth RA, Greer SL, Albert JM, Young EW, Piette JD. Out-of-pocket spending and medication adherence among dialysis patients in twelve countries. *Health Aff (Millwood).* 2008;27:89-102.

17. Piette JD, Heisler M, Wagner TH. Cost-related medication under-use among chronically ill adults: what treatments do people forego? How often? Who is at risk? *Am J Public Health.* 2004;94:1782-7.

18. Piette JD, Wagner TH, Potter MB, Schillinger D. Health insurance status, cost-related medication underuse, and outcomes among diabetes patients in three systems of care. *Med Care.* 2004;42:102-9.

19. National Institute for Health and Clinical Excellence (NICE). [28 Jan 2009]. Medicines Adherence: Involving patients in decisions about prescribed medicines and supporting adherence (CG76): NICE Guideline 76. Available from: http://guidance.nice.org.uk/CG76.

20. Karamanidou C, Weinman J, Horne R. Improving haemodialysis patients' understanding of phosphate binding medication: a pilot study of a psycho-educational intervention designed to change patients' perceptions of the problem and treatment. *Brit J Health Psychol.* 2008;13:205-14.

21. Berry DC, Knapp P, Raynor DK. Provision of information about drug side-effects to patients. *Lancet.* 2002;359:853-4.

22. Bowskill R, Clatworthy J, Parham R, Rank T, Horne R. Patients' perceptions of information received about medication prescribed for bipolar disorder: Implications for informed choice. *J Affect Disord.* 2007;100:253-7.

23. Gellaitry G, Cooper V, Davis C, Fisher M, Date HL, Horne R. Patients' perception of information about HAART: impact on treatment decisions. *AIDS Care.* 2005;17:367-76.

24. Horne R, Hankins M, Jenkins R. The satisfaction with information about medicines scale (SIMS): a new measurement tool for audit and research. *Qual Health Care.* 2001;10: 135-40.

25. Raynor DK, Britten N. Medicine information leaflets fail concordance test. *BMJ.* 2001;322:1541.

26. Dickinson D, Raynor DK. What information do patients need about medicines? Ask the patients—they may want to know more than you think. *BMJ.* 2003;327:861.

27. Clifford S, Barber N, Horne R. The difference in medication-related beliefs held by adherers, intentional non-adherers and unintentional non-adherers. Paper presented at the oral presentation at the annual conference of the BPS Division of Health Psychology. 2006.

28. Emilsson MB, Berndtsson I, Lötvall J, Millqvist E, Lundgren J, Johansson A, et al. The influence of personality traits and beliefs about medicines on adherence to asthma treatment. *Prim Care Respir J.* 2011;20:141-7.

29. Horne R. Compliance, adherence and concordance. In: Taylor K, Harding G, editors. Pharmacy practice. London: Taylor and Francis; 2001. p. 165-84.

30. Horne R. Adherence to asthma medication: a question of ability? *Prim Care Respir J.* 2011;20:118-9.

31. Horne R, Weinman J. Patients' beliefs about prescribed medicines and their role in adherence to treatment in chronic physical illness. *J Psychosom Res.* 1999;47:555-67.

32. Horne R, Weinman J. Self-regulation and self-management in asthma: exploring the role of illness perceptions and treatment beliefs in explaining non-adherence to preventer medication. *Psychol Health.* 2002;17:17-32.

33. Horne R, Weinman J, Hankins M. The Beliefs about Medicines Questionnaire: the development and evaluation of a new method for assessing the cognitive representation of medication. *Psychol Health.* 1999;14:1-24.

34. Menckeberg TT, Bouvy ML, Bracke M, Kaptein AA, Leufkens HG, Raaijmakers JA, et al. Beliefs about medicines predict refill adherence to inhaled corticosteroids. *J Psychosom Res.* 2008;64:47-54.

35. Tibaldi G, Clatworthy J, Torchio E, Argentero P, Munizza C, Horne R. The utility of the Necessity—Concerns Framework in explaining treatment non-adherence in four chronic illness groups in Italy. *Chronic Illn.* 2009;5:129-33.

36. Horne R. Treatment perceptions and self regulation. In: Cameron LD, Leventhal H, editors. The self-regulation of health and illness behaviour. London: Routledge; 2003. p. 138-53.

37. Clatworthy J, Price D, Ryan D, Haughney J, Horne R. The value of self-report assessment of adherence, rhinitis and smoking in relation to asthma control. *Prim Care Respir J.* 2009;18:300-5.

38. Leventhal H, Brissette I, Leventhal E. The common-sense model of self-regulation of health and illness. In: Cameron LD, Leventhal H, editors. The self-regulation of health and illness behaviour. NY: Routledge; 2003. p. 42.

39. Leventhal H, Leventhal E, Cameron L. Representations, procedures, and affect in illness self-regulation: a perceptual-cognitive model. In: Baum A, Revenson TA, Singer J, editors. Handbook of health psychology. New Jersey: Pergamon Press; 2001. p. 19.

40. Halm EA, Mora P, Leventhal H. No symptoms, no asthma: the acute episodic disease belief is associated with poor self-management among inner-city adults with persistent asthma. *Chest.* 2006;129:573-80.

41. Calnan M, Montaner D, Horne R. How acceptable are innovative health-care technologies? A survey of public beliefs and attitudes in England and Wales. *Soc Sci Med.* 2005;60:1937-48.

42. Horne R. Compliance, adherence, and concordance: implications for asthma treatment. *Chest.* 2006;130:65S-72S.

43. Cooper V, Gellaitry G, Horne R. Treatment perceptions and self-regulation in adherence to HAART. *Int J Behav Med.* 2004;11:81.

44. Siegel K, Dean L, Schrimshaw E. Symptom ambiguity among late middle aged and older adults with HIV. *Res Aging.* 1999;21:595-618.

45. Bulloch AG, Adair CE, Patten SB. Forgetfulness: a role in noncompliance with antidepressant treatment. *Can J Psychiatry.* 2006;51:719-22.

46. Franks TJ, Burton DL, Simpson MD. Patient medication knowledge and adherence to asthma pharmacotherapy: a pilot study in rural Australia. *Ther Clin Risk Manag.* 2005;1:33-8.

47. Woods SP, Dawson MS, Weber E, Gibson S, Grant I, Atkinson JH. Timing is everything: antiretroviral nonadherence is associated with impairment in time-based prospective memory. *J Int Neuropsychol Soc.* 2009;15:42-52.

48. Wadsworth E, Normal P, Searle A, Mitchell J, Macrae N, O'Mahony M, et al. Habitual prospective memory in elderly patients with type 2 diabetes: implications for medication adherence. *Psychol Health Med.* 2004;9:17-27.

49. Incalzi RA, Gemma A, Marra C, Capparella O, Fuso L, Carbonin P. Verbal memory impairment in COPD: its mechanisms and clinical relevance. *Chest.* 1997;112:1506-13.

50. Vincent EC, Hardin PA, Norman LA, Lester EA, Stinton SH. The effects of a computer-assisted reminder system on patient compliance with recommended health maintenance procedures. *Proc Annu Symp Comput Appl Med Care.* 1995;656-60.

51. Wise J, Operario D. Use of electronic reminder devices to improve adherence to antiretroviral therapy: a systematic review. *AIDS Patient Care STDS.* 2008;22:495-504.

52. Gollwitzer PM. Goal achievement: the role of intentions. *Eur Rev Social Psychol.* 1993;4:141-85.

53. Brown I, Sheeran P, Reuber M. Enhancing antiepileptic drug adherence: a randomized controlled trial. *Epilepsy Behav.* 2009;16:634-9.

54. DiMatteo MR, Lepper HS, Croghan TW. Depression is a risk factor for noncompliance with medical treatment: meta-analysis of the effects of anxiety and depression on patient adherence. *Arch Intern Med.* 2000;160:2101-7.

55. Nunes V, Neilson J, O'Flynn N, Calvert N, Kuntze S, Smithson H, et al. Clinical Guidelines and Evidence Review for Medicines Adherence: involving patients in decisions about prescribed medicines and supporting adherence. 2009. Available from http://www.nice.org.uk/nicemedia/pdf/CG76NICEGuideline.pdf.

56. Clifford S, Barber N, Elliott R, Hartley E, Horne R. Patient centred advice is effective in improving adherence to medicines. *Pharm World Sci.* 2006;28:165-70.

57. Gamble J Stevenson M, Heaney LG. A study of a multi-level intervention to improve non-adherence in difficult to control asthma. *Respir Med.* 2011;105:1308-15.

58. Cohen J, Mann D, Wisnivesky J, Leventhal H, Horne R, Musumeci-Szabó T, et al. Assessing the validity of self-reported medication adherence among inner-city asthmatic adults: The Medication Adherence Reporting Scale for Asthma. *Ann Allergy Asthma Immunol.* 2009;103:325-31.

59. De Bruin M, Hopsers HJ, Van Den Borne HW, Kok G, Prins JM. Theory and evidence-based intervention to improve adherence to antiretroviral therapy among HIV-infected patients in the Netherlands:A pilot study. *AIDS Patient Care STDs.* 2005;19:384-94.

60. Woodruff PG, Modrek B, Choy DF, Jia G, Abbas AR, Ellwanger A, et al. T-helper type 2-driven inflammation defines major subphenotypes of asthma. *Am J Respir Crit Care Med.* 2009;180:388-95.

61. Global Strategy for Asthma Management and Prevention, Global Initiative for Asthma (GINA) 2010. Available from: http://www.ginasthma.org

62. British Thoracic Society Scottish Intercollegiate Guidelines Network. British Guideline on the Management of Asthma. *Thorax.* 2008;63:iv1-121.

Psychological Morbidity in Difficult-to-treat Asthma

Adel H Mansur, Alison Pooler

INTRODUCTION

In a difficult asthma clinic, psychology, in many ways, plays a critical role in the patient's disease presentation and level of morbidity. Difficult asthma patients often display increased levels of anxiety, depression, or other forms of psychological distress. Anxious and depressed asthmatics have worse asthma control measures and utilize higher level of medical resources when compared to those with normal anxiety or depression parameters. Coping strategies of an individual with severe asthma and depression are impaired and relate to asthma exacerbation frequency and severity.

The existence of personality disorders, certain behavioral attitudes, and psychiatric diseases in an asthmatic confound his/her management and asthma control. Chronic hyperventilation syndromes, panic syndromes, and vocal cord dysfunction coexist or are misdiagnosed as asthma and are associated with morbid psychologies. These include traumatic childhood experiences, physical and sexual abuse, and adverse psychosocial conditions. Some patients exaggerate asthma symptoms for a variety of reasons.

Undiagnosed associated psychological factors undermine asthma treatment. In any difficult asthma clinic, a full understanding of the psychological aspects of asthma and associated syndromes is critical for making the correct diagnosis and institution of appropriate management plans. This chapter discusses the levels of psychological distress, rates of psychiatric disorders, personality disorders, coping styles, role of a psychologist, and psychological interventions in a difficult asthma clinic.

HISTORICAL PERSPECTIVE (ASTHMA NERVOSA)

The concept of asthma nervosa goes a long way back in history, with more interest seen during the renaissance period.[1] In the 1750s, an English physician and actor, John Hill, suggested that effective remedies, such as spring honey taken regularly and sometimes in conjunction with a perennial herb, *Erysimum*, cured asthmatic fits and prevented their return, but he primarily considered asthma as a nervous complaint.[2] George Cheyne (1671–1743) also regarded asthma as one of the range of modern "nervous distempers."[3] William Cullen (Scottish surgeon, 1710–1790) developed interest in the central role played by the disorders of the nervous system in disease causation (adopting a neuropathological approach). This approach was linked to the wider enlightenment anxieties about the impact of modern civilization on health.[4] Cullen related the apparent rise of chronic nervous diseases to the greater sensibility of Western-civilized nations, caused partly by constitutional factors, such as race, class, gender, and age, and partly by luxurious and sedentary lifestyles. Cullen's explanation of the causes of asthma and related "nervous conditions" (such as hysteria, hypochondria, dyspepsia, and gout) had an important impact on perceiving asthma as a nervous disorder. Cullen's classification of asthma as a form of neurosis and his perception of its effective treatment was extended and published in a full length treatise by Thomas Withers (1750–1809), a physician at the York County Hospital UK, who described the cause of asthma as a "violent passion of the mind."[5]

The early 20th century's discovery of allergy and its link to asthma did not undermine the perceived connection between asthma and the mind. The two theories of asthma were often explored in tandem. Initial studies of the psychogenic aspects of asthma were often carried out in allergy clinics and tended to merge psychological and immunological approaches to the disease. Clinical studies on both sides of the Atlantic continued to emphasize the emotional determinants of asthma. In UK, during the 1920's, Arthur Hurst and Humphrey Rolleston explored cases of "hysterical and emotional asthma" in which an "irritable bronchial center" was stimulated not only by a familiar array of physical irritants, but by psychological factors, such as excitement and worry.[6,7] A German physician, Erich Wittkower (1899–1983) described the typical allergy patient as a delicate, upper-class only child who developed into a socially and emotionally maladjusted adult.[8] In North America, Horace Baldwin (1895–1983) suggested that asthma attacks could be triggered by strain, fatigue, depression, and worry brought on by caring for sick relatives, family arguments, or marital problems.[9] A Scottish physician, James Lorimer Halliday (1897–1983), regarded asthma as "a bodily manifestation of emotional reaction," usually precipitated in the first instance by a perceived threat to life.[10]

In the inter-war years, psychosomatic medicine developed further on the basis of Freudian psychoanalysis and the physiological studies of emotions carried out by Walter Cannon. According to Dunbar, the asthmatic wheeze constituted the "suppressed cry" of a patient suffocated by an over attentive mother. It was believed that asthma could be traced to a traumatic childhood.[11] Indeed, there are theories that type I brittle asthma has its origins in childhood trauma and abuse.[12]

Historically, therefore, asthma has long been considered a psychosomatic illness in which changes in mood and emotions play a major role in symptom presentation.[13] Psychosomatic illnesses are often now referred to as psychophysiological disorders, which convey the idea that the mind (psych) is having an undesirable effect on the body (soma).[14] This is often referred to as psychological factors.

ASTHMA PSYCHOPATHOLOGY

There is a substantial body of evidence to support the role of complex neural mechanisms, altered autonomic nervous system control, and neural-immune pathways in the pathophysiology and symptomatology of asthma.[15-17] The autonomic nervous system can regulate airway caliber and function through effects on airway smooth muscle, bronchial vessels, and mucus glands. Hormones and neuropeptides released into the circulation when individuals experience stress are also thought to be involved in regulating both inflammatory and airway responses.[18] Stress through altered regulation of the hypothalamic-pituitary-adrenal and sympathetic-adrenomedullary axes may have immunomodulatory effects on atopy favoring type 2 helper T cell (Th2) biased response favoring allergic outcomes.[19] The field of psychoneuroimmunology links psychosocial stress, the central nervous system, and alterations in immune and endocrine functions and provides plausible biological understanding linking the brain to asthma presentation and its severity.

There is evidence of a causal bidirectional relationship between asthma and psychosocial factors both in development and prognosis of asthma. Emotional stress, anxiety, and post-traumatic stress disorders seem to precede development of asthma in children and adults.[20] Asthma precedes panic disorders and panic disorders may exacerbate preexisting asthma.[21] In a meta-analysis of 43 prospective cohort studies, Chida et al. investigated the influence of psychosocial factors on atopic disorders (asthma 90.7%, rhinitis 4.7%, dermatitis 2.3%, and food allergies 2.3%) and the effect of such atopic disorders on mental health.[22] This revealed a positive association between psychosocial factors and future atopic disorder development, as well as between the presence of atopic disorders and poor future mental health. The subgroup meta-analysis on the healthy and atopic disorder populations showed that psychosocial factors had both an etiological and prognostic effect on atopic disorders.

The prevalence of anxiety disorders in asthmatic population is increased, but not all asthma patients are anxious. In addition, while there is some evidence to support that anxiety is more common in patients with more severe asthma symptoms, this does not explain the extent to which asthma severity may act as a primary cause of anxiety. It is, therefore, likely that other factors, besides asthma severity, play a role in the development and maintenance of anxiety disorders, which would explain why some patients worry more about their condition than other patients. The Clark's cognitive model of anxiety/panic in asthma (Figure 5-1) proposes that panic attacks occur when individuals perceive certain somatic sensations as considerably more dangerous than they truly are, and then they interpret them to mean that they are

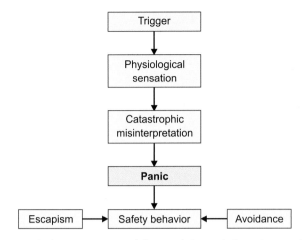

Figure 5-1 Clark's cognitive model to explain panic in asthma patients.[23]

about to experience sudden, imminent disaster.[23] The vicious circle ending in a panic attack develops when a stimulus perceived as threatening creates a feeling of anxiety. Therefore, if the somatic sensations that accompany this state of anxiety are catastrophically misinterpreted, the individual starts to experience a further increase in anxiety, followed by elevated somatic sensations until a full blown panic attack occurs. Maladaptive cognitive appraisals enhance anxiety, which will inevitably lead to a panic attack. Unpleasant past incidents of experiencing a panic attack will produce memory biases and anxious individuals show a tendency to pay specific attention to threatening stimuli, which serve as a major concern for them. Anxious people display low self-efficacy, and as a result their perception of personal inability to control their anxiety symptoms under a harmful situation will lead them to escapism, behavioral avoidance, and safety seeking behavior.[24]

The answer to the question of why asthma is associated with depression is uncertain. The prevalent notion is that reduced functioning and quality of life, secondary to chronic illness, leads to depression.[25] In an inner-city study, 85 adults with asthma and concomitant major depressive disorder had mean age of onset of 21 and 28.8 years, respectively. Asthma preceded depression in 62% of cases, depression preceded asthma in 24% of cases, and asthma and depression had concurrent onset in 14% of cases, suggesting that depression generally occurs after asthma.[26] The other possibility for this relationship is the presence of undiscovered biological factors (e.g., genetic disposition), which increase susceptibility to both disorders. Dysregulation of cholinergic pathways has been implicated in both depression and asthma.[27] Increases in airway constriction, which may be mediated by cholinergic pathways, are associated with stress or negative mood states in asthma patients.[28-30]

IMPACT OF PSYCHOLOGICAL AND PSYCHIATRIC COMORBIDITY IN ASTHMA

Stress/Anxiety and Depression

The main psychological and psychiatric disorders associated with asthma are stress/anxiety and depression. Depression and anxiety appear to be more common in people with asthma, than in general population,[13] and stress and anxiety are thought to be important factors in instigating or contributing to asthma exacerbations in some individuals.

Depressive symptoms and depressive disorders are common in medical settings.[31] When present in medically ill patients, depression appears to be associated with further decrease in the ability to carry out daily activities and quality of life.[5] Depression seems to be common in patients with asthma,[32] and studies have shown that in patients with asthma, there are both higher levels of prevalence and more severe levels of depression than in healthy subjects.[33,34] Depression may also have adverse effects on asthma. Several reports suggest that depression may be a risk factor for asthma-related morbidity and mortality.[35,36]

Studies of asthma and anxiety disorders in adults have predominantly focused on examining the relationship between asthma symptoms and severity of asthma, and anxiety symptoms and markers of asthma, such as breathlessness.[37] The finding that asthma and anxiety disorders coexist at a rate greater than expected by chance is critical for treatment planning and decision making, especially if comorbid anxiety disorders result in poorer prognosis of asthma, because efficacious treatments for anxiety disorders are available, as outlined in the anxiety management guidelines.[38] From a population perspective, the link between asthma and anxiety disorders has considerable public health importance. The prevalence of asthma rose by more than threefold in the past two decades. However, anxiety disorders are widely under recognized, under diagnosed, and under treated in general medical and community settings.[13] Majority of studies examining the relationship between asthma and anxiety disorders in adults have reported significant associations between the two conditions.[33,39,40] Kolbe et al. observed a considerable increase in general psychological morbidity and anxiety in patients admitted to hospital with acute asthma, as compared to a community based control group.[41] Greaves et al. found that anxiety was more common in patients who had suffered a recent exacerbation than those with well-controlled asthma.[42] In the latter study, a patient's psychological reaction to an asthma attack seemed to predict whether she/he will require future emergency care for asthma. Overall, patients with recent asthma attacks had higher panic and anxiety scores and lower confidence scores than the control group. They were also more likely to have been treated for anxiety and depression in the last three years.

These studies collectively confirm the notion of increased levels of anxiety and depression in asthma, particularly following an acute asthma attack. The presence of depression or anxiety is likely to impair an asthmatic's ability to manage his/her asthma, particularly to self-medicate and self-manage when faced with an acute attack. These studies have yielded the need for recognition and treatment of anxiety and depression as comorbidities in asthma.

It must be realized, however, that many conditions may mimic asthma or aspects of asthma and some of these mimickers are psychosomatic in aetiology, for example, hyperventilation syndromes, psychogenic cough, and vocal cord dysfunction.[43-47] Intriguingly, anxiety symptoms in patients have been shown to be strong predictors of the misdiagnosis of asthma.[48]

Asthma Death/Near-fatal Asthma Studies

A number of retrospective confidential enquiries and case-control studies of asthma deaths have reported an association between psychosocial factors and patients who die from asthma.[49-51] In a UK study of 533 cases of fatal asthma and 533 matched controls (hospital admissions in the same geographical region), 75% of cases had a prior recorded psychological factor as compared to 79% of controls, suggesting that psychology affects hospital admission rather than asthma deaths.[52] In another study of near-fatal asthma, 77 cases 293 controls (hospital admissions) were compared to 100 community-based asthmatic control group. The level of psychological morbidity in the near-fatal and hospital admission groups was similar and higher than the community controls.[41] The levels of psychological morbidity reported in this study were substantially lower than the levels reported in 'out-patients' with severe asthma. Intriguingly, "as in many fatal/near-fatal asthma studies," 32–44% of patients in each group were not on inhaled steroids. This reflects the fact that in fatal or near-fatal asthma, significant proportion of patients do not fulfill any definition of severe or 'difficult to control' asthma.

Studies in Severe Asthma

In a case/control study of type I 'brittle asthma' (a condition characterized by chaotic changes in peak flow on background of severe asthma with propensity to rapid severe attacks), psychological morbidity (using the General Health Questionnaire and Living with Asthma Questionnaire) was significantly elevated compared to controls of non-brittle asthma.[53] In difficult-to-treat asthma, using a structured protocol to assess the prevalence of comorbidities, two observational UK studies reported high levels of comorbidity and suggested that up to 50% of subjects evaluated in a difficult asthma clinic do not have refractory/therapy resistant disease. These studies reported high levels of psychological morbidity in this broad difficult asthma population. In the Belfast study of 73 sequentially referred subjects,

50% had a psychiatric diagnosis after formal psychiatric interview (the diagnostic gold standard).[54,55] Of these, in 27 of 32 subjects (84%), psychiatric diagnosis had not been previously identified, and depression was the most common diagnosis, observed in 19 out of 73 subjects (29%). In the Brompton study, using pre-agreed definitions, which attempted to relate asthma symptoms to psychological symptoms, of 56 subjects evaluated, 58% were felt to have a 'psychiatric contribution' to their asthma.[56] Pooler found that the prevalence of depression in severe asthma was 44%, of which 16% were labelled as severe, as measured by the Hospital Anxiety and Depression Score (HADS). In the latter study, severe depression led to more severe and frequent asthma exacerbations. In addition, 48% of the severe asthmatics in this study displayed increased HADS scores for anxiety, but none received any treatment or management for their anxiety states.[57]

Data from these studies collectively confirm high prevalence of psychological co-morbidity (depression and anxiety, in particular) in the difficult and severe asthma settings. This psychological comorbidity tends to be under-recognized and under treated.

Personality Factors, Attitudes, Beliefs, and Coping Styles

Personality traits represent habitual patterns of behavior, thought, and emotion that are far more enduring and chronic than acute experiences of psychological distress, and more persistent than psychiatric disorders. The persistent and independent nature of certain personality traits may make asthma difficult to treat through their potential to interfere with disease self-management and the patient's willingness to seek and/or accept treatment. Chetta et al. studied masculinity/femininity, depressive, paranoid, social introversion, and hypochondrias personality traits using the Minnesota multipahsic personality inventory in 36 patients with various degree of asthma severity. In the moderate to severe asthma group, there was higher overall prevalence of personality disorders, hypochondriasis, and poorer perception of breathlessness than in the mild asthma group.[58] Different study revealed increased prevalence of alexithymia in 19 near-fatal asthmatics when compared to 19 non-near-fatal asthmatics, but other specific personality profiles were similar in both groups.[59] The dimensions of personality (such as novelty seeking, harm avoidance, reward dependence, persistence, and self directedness) amongst 90 severe and 37 mild asthmatics did not differ in another study.[60]

Attitudes and beliefs can influence how an individual copes with asthma. In a study of 137 patients admitted to hospital with severe asthma, pessimism and concerns about disease-related stigma were associated with less asthma knowledge and poorer self-management behavior.[61] Other studies could not confirm relation between attitudes/beliefs and asthma severity[41] or patients knowledge and asthma severity.[62] Patients with more external and/or less internal locus of control are thought to be at higher risk of worse asthma outcomes, since those who believe that they could not control their disease may be less likely to engage in self-management. Severe asthmatics appear to have lower external locus of control beliefs relative to mild asthma, however, difficult-to-treat asthmatics show higher external locus of control beliefs relative to well-controlled asthmatics.[60,63] This may explain in part the high prevalence of poor treatment adherence in difficult-to-treat asthma.

Denial attitudes were linked to asthma deaths in 8–14% of cases in two studies,[49,50] which could be related to patients failing to accept severity of their illness and act properly in terms of treatment adherence and seeking timely help. Patients may delay seeking treatment during acute exacerbations and these delays have been associated with psychological factors such as panic and stressful life events.[64] A comprehensive assessment of emotional-cognitive and behavioral styles in asthma using the Millon Behavioural Medicine Diagnostic Inventory showed that patients with severe asthma vs. moderate asthma had significantly higher scores for illness apprehension, pessimism, and interventional fragility.[65] Pessimistic patients with negative attitudes are less likely to attend and follow treatments, leading to worse asthma outcome and impaired quality of life.

In conclusion, there is some evidence for a role of personality traits (hypochondriasis and alexithymia), beliefs and attitudes (e.g., pessimism and locus of control), and coping styles (e.g., denial and treatment avoidance) in severe asthma morbidity. However, there is a clear need for further research to establish this role.

Factitious Disease "Asthma"

In a difficult asthma clinic setting, factitious disease (FD) "presenting as asthma" (Munchausen syndrome) poses a difficult challenge to physicians in terms of making the diagnosis in first place and the subsequent management. While clinicians working in this field will all have experienced some patients with this diagnosis, research into the prevalence of this condition in the difficult asthma clinic, and how to make the diagnosis has not been done. The word factitious asthma has been used to describe other entities such as vocal cord dysfunction (VCD). However, this should not be the case as VCD is an entirely different disease. Three criteria need to be met for diagnosis of FD. These include intentional production of physical or psychological signs or symptoms, motivation for the behavior is to assume the sick role, and absence of external incentives for the behavior (e.g., economic gain, avoiding legal responsibility, improving physical well-being, as in malingering).[66] Three types of FD described include those with predominantly psychological signs and symptoms, predominantly physical signs and symptoms, and combined psychological and physical signs and symptoms.

Patients with factitious asthma may in the outset appear to have some subjective measures suggestive of an asthma diagnosis including presence of symptoms of wheeze, tightness, and breathlessness. However, closer examination employing physiological testing including bronchial provocation and airway inflammation measures will not be positive. A pattern of repeated admissions and need for high cost-investigations and treatments is common. Often, there is a feeling of helplessness by the clinical team in terms of controlling symptoms or admission frequency. Episodes of endotracheal intubation/ventilation and intensive care treatment may be observed but characteristically airway and inflation pressure would be normal and such episodes will be brief.[67,68] Previous reports of FD observed increased prevalence in young females, who may have worked in nursing or other allied healthcare professions, while patients with chronic FD tend to be middle-aged males.[69] FD should be distinguished from other somatoform disorders and malingering. In case of somatoform disorders, production of symptoms of illness is not intentional, and motivation for illness is unconscious; in FD, symptoms are produced intentionally but for unconscious reasons; and in malingering, symptom production is intentional and conscious to achieve an external incentive beyond assuming the sick role (for example, evading the police, obtaining sick benefit or disability allowances, social hospital admission, etc). In practice, however, determining whether an external incentive exists can sometimes be difficult. Additionally, in practice, FD behavior could present in patients with clear cut asthma, a situation that poses most of the challenge to clinicians in terms of dissecting what is a true disease from an aberrant behavior.

Psychological Effects of Systemic Corticosteroids

A survey of UK difficult asthma clinics showed that 40% of patients were on long-term maintenance steroids therapy, receiving a mean dose of predsnisolone or equivalent of 15 mg/day.[70] Corticosteroids-related side effects are significant causes of increased morbidity associated with difficult asthma. However, while the somatic side effects of corticosteroid therapy are well recognized and generally receive good attention, neuropsychiatric side effects are often ignored and not explored. This is surprising given the fact that this population has increased psychological morbidity which potentially may be aggravated by concomitant corticosteroid treatment.

Corticosteroid therapy alone, in the short-term (less than one month of treatment duration), has been linked with various psychiatric side effects. Two meta-analyses found that severe psychiatric reactions occurred in nearly 6% of patients, and mild-to-moderate reactions occurred in about 28%.[71,72] Although disturbances of mood, cognition, sleep, and behavior, as well as frank delirium or even psychosis are possible, most common adverse effects of short-term corticosteroid therapy are euphoria and hypomania.[73]

Long-term corticosteroid therapy tends to induce depressive symptoms. Dosage seems to relate directly to the incidence of adverse effects, but not to the timing, severity, or duration of these effects. In outpatients receiving prednisone therapy (7.5 mg/d for 6 months) and similar controls, current mood was evaluated using the Hamilton Rating Scale for Depression (HRSD), Young Mania Rating Scale, Brief Psychiatric Rating Scale, Internal State Scale, and a diagnostic interview. Twelve (60%) of 20 corticosteroid-treated patients met diagnostic criteria for a lifetime prednisone-induced mood disorder. This study showed predominant depressive rather than manic symptoms based on clinician-rated assessments.[74] History of previous reactions does not predict adverse responses to subsequent courses of corticosteroids. Corticosteroid-induced symptoms frequently present early in a treatment cycle and typically resolve with dosage reduction or discontinuation of corticosteroids. In severe cases or situations in which the dose cannot be reduced, antipsychotics or mood stabilizers may be required. In an open label-controlled clinical trial, olanzapine was well tolerated and appears to be useful for treating mood disturbances associated with corticosteroid therapy.[75]

Cognitive impairment, particularly in the form of memory deficits has been observed in both long- and short-term corticosteroid therapy. Deficits during short-term therapy are consistent with hippocampal dysfunction and occur with reversible atrophy of hippocampal neurons.[76,77] These disturbances appear to be dose dependent and reversible with corticosteroid discontinuation. Cognitive/ memory deficits may interfere with the ability to undertake self-management plans and general treatment concordance in asthma. This notion has generally received little attention in the difficult asthma clinics and requires further research to identify its extent and any links to adverse clinical outcomes.

TREATMENT OF MORBID PSYCHOLOGY IN DIFFICULT ASTHMA

Anxiety and Depression

NICE has developed guidelines for the management of anxiety and depression in primary and secondary care.[78] Within these guidelines one of the key priorities is for implementation of screening to be undertaken in primary and secondary care for anxiety and depression in high-risk groups, such as people with a chronic disease like severe or difficult asthma.

Many people with an established chronic disease become depressed or anxious during the course of their illness, and recognition and treatment of such comorbidity can lead to increased quality of life. When reviewing the literature, there are several psychological interventions that are considered appropriate to reduce psychological problems associated with asthma. These include behavioral therapies, cognitive therapies, cognitive behavioral therapy (CBT), relaxation techniques, psychodynamic psychotherapies, and counseling for individuals and groups. The aim of these therapies is to influence the patient by psychological means so that their symptoms decrease or there is a positive change in behavior. They also aim to help reduce panic or fear, improve breathing and respiratory function, and impact positively on general health and quality of life.

When managing patients, clinical staff need to have reliable information on whether psychological techniques work, and if so, which are the most effective for which patients? It is also important to know whether interventions work best alone or in combination and in individual or group sessions. Despite this, psychological interventions receive little or no mention in international guidelines, such as the BTS/SIGN or GINA asthma guidelines.

Does the Treatment of Psychological Comorbidities Alter Asthma Outcomes?

There is no available robust evidence to support the use of psychological interventions for patients with severe and difficult asthma, or even asthma of any severity. A systematic review, which examined the evidence for psychological interventions for adults with asthma, could not draw any firm conclusions about the effectiveness of such interventions due to the poor quality of the included studies, insufficient data reporting, and the varied outcome measures utilized.[79] The psychological interventions themselves were also varied without clear underpinning theory to their application in such clinical settings. The only positive results that were drawn, although not totally conclusive, showed improvement of quality of life following CBT. A meta-analysis of psychoeducational interventions in difficult asthma concluded that studies were of poor quality, with some evidence of positive effect of psychosocial educational interventions on hospital admissions and asthma symptoms in adults and children, but not enough evidence to warrant significant changes in clinical practice and little information available on cost effectiveness.[80] The same group performed a non-blinded randomized intervention study in adults using a broad definition of 'difficult asthma' and showed no benefit from a 6-month nurse-delivered psychoeducational program.[81] The wide definition of difficult asthma used in the latter study, the lack of a precise psychiatric diagnosis, and the generic nonspecific intervention (i.e., the intervention was the same for all patients) were possible causes for the negative outcome. Interestingly, when a single psychiatric disease is targeted, an important proof of concept study suggested that there may be some benefit.[82] This study examined the effect of citalopram or placebo (12 weeks) in 82 subjects with depression (diagnosed using the HRSD, a 21 multiple choice questionnaire that rates the severity of a patient's depressive illness) and asthma. A reduction in depressive symptoms was associated with improvement in asthma control and corticosteroid use for severe asthma exacerbations in the citalopram group. However, by inference the severity of asthma in the study population seems to be mild-to-moderate.

There is a clear lack of an evidence base for psychological interventions in difficult-to-treat asthma, largely due to the paucity of quality controlled clinical trials, which prompts an urgent need to conduct much needed further research in this area. As it stands, giving the high psychological burden in difficult-to-treat asthma, the effectiveness of any psychological intervention needs to be monitored closely to prove its worth and safety in any individual.

ROLE OF A PSYCHOLOGIST IN A DIFFICULT ASTHMA CLINIC

Psychological factors influence outcomes in difficult asthma and should be properly assessed (Figure 5-2). A psychologist's role within a difficult asthma clinic setting is seen as being increasingly essential. One of the main aims of a psychologist is to assess for the presence of any important psychological/psychiatric factors, the impact of such psychiatric disease or distress level on the patient's asthma symptoms, and the way such a patient adapts to his/her illness. This should allow for an individualized stepwise management program aiming at addressing and treating any underlying psychiatric illness (e.g., depression), and managing asthma-related issues, such as improving adherence and disease coping strategies or reducing stress levels. The ability to conduct CBT is an important component of any such service. For a psychologist to be effective in the management of difficult asthma, she/he has to develop an indepth understanding of the causes of difficult asthma and related comorbidities and other specifics in terms of asthma management. The ability to engage and establish rapport and gain confidence of such patients who may be wary "because of difficult life experiences" to open-up or engage is an essential skill for the psychologist. Awareness of difficult presentations, including traumatic childhood experience, including physical or sexual abuse or other domestic violence is required. A psychologist should have skills to address behavioral issues, such as the "sick role" and hidden gains from disease, or even factitious asthma, which can be very challenging. The ability of a psychologist to develop an indepth understanding of difficult asthma, establish rapport and effectively engage patients, diagnose their needs, and act in an effective way to change behavior are the essential ingredients for a successful psychologist, which in our experience is an essential component of any difficult asthma service.

Psychologists within a difficult asthma clinic need to work within a multi-disciplinary team. They have a role in educating the larger team and may even train some team members to develop skills in recognizing psychological distress, psychiatric disease, personality disorders, and management of challenging personalities. This multidisciplinary role is important for the wider team to improve its effectiveness to interact with difficult asthma patients and improve overall satisfaction and patient experience.

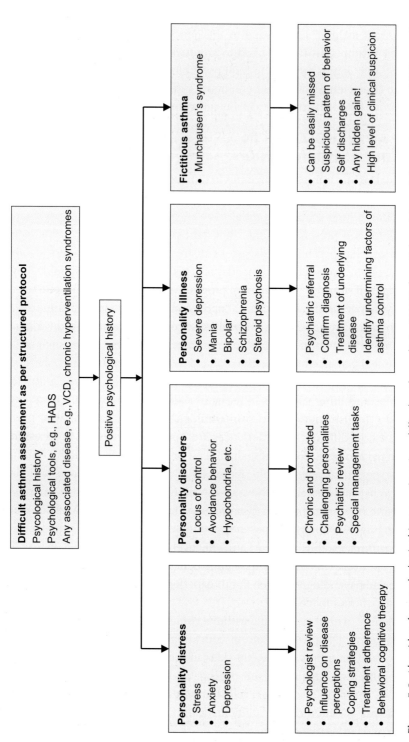

Figure 5-2 Algorithm for psychological interventions in a difficult asthma clinic. HADS, hospital anxiety and depression score; VCD, vocal cord dysfunction.

FUTURE RESEARCH

As illustrated in figure 5-2, while the morbid psychology in a difficult asthma clinic setting is obvious and likely to play a significant part in patient outcomes related to asthma or otherwise, the evidence base for how best to set up clinical practice in terms of patients' screening, diagnosis, and treatment is lacking. Future research should focus on the following areas to complete existing knowledge gaps:

- Accurate estimate of psychological burden in severe/difficult-to-treat asthma
- Definition of the psychological/psychiatric disease spectrum in a difficult asthma clinic
- Determination of clinical and cost effectiveness of psychological intervention in improving general quality of life and asthma outcomes
- Establishing best clinical practice to effectively manage psychological comorbidities within a difficult asthma clinic.

REFERENCES

1. Jackson M. Asthma: the biography. New York: Oxford University Press, 2009.
2. Hill J. The Virtue of Honey. London: 1759: 4, p. 26-31.
3. Cheyne G. The English Malady. London: 1733. p. 226-37.
4. Cullen W. First Line of Practice of Physic, iii. (Edinburgh 1783), 390.
5. Wells KB, Stewart A, Hays RD, Burnam MA, Rogers W, Daniels M, Berry S, Greenfield S, Withers T. *A Treatise on Asthma*. London; 1786. p. vii-viii.
6. Hurst AF. An Address On Asthma. *Lancet*. 1921;1:1113-7.
7. Rolleston H. Idiosyncrasies. London; 1927. p. 92-102.
8. Wittkower E. Studies in hay fever patients "the allergic personality". *J Ment Sci*. 1938; 84:352-69.
9. Horace S, Baldwin. 'Studies in the asthmatic state: I. The stimulus' *J Allergy*. 1929;1:124-9.
10. Halliday JL. Approach to asthma. *Br Med J*. 1937;17:1-53.
11. Dunbar F. Mind and body: Psychosomatic medicine. *New York*. 1947:177.
12. Ayres JG, Miles JF, Barnes PJ. Brittle Asthma. *Thorax*. 1998;53:315-21.
13. Brown ES (ed): Asthma: Social and Psychological Factors and Psychosomatic Syndromes. *Adv Psychosom Med*. 2003;24:131-60.
14. Kring AM, Davison GC, Neale JM, Johnson SL. Abnormal Psychology. New 10th ed Jersey: John Wiley and sons Ltd; 2007.
15. Barnes PJ. Airway inflammation and autonomic control. *Eur J Respir Dis Suppl*. 1986; 147:80-7.
16. Barnes PJ. Is asthma a nervous disease? *Chest*. 1995;107:119S-125S.
17. Barnes PJ. Overview of neural mechanisms in asthma. *Pulm Pharmacol*. 1995;8:151-9.
18. Moran MG. Psychological factors affecting pulmonary and rheumatologic diseases. A review. *Psychosomatics*. 1991;32:14-23.
19. Haczku A, Panettieri RA Jr. Social stress and asthma: the role of corticosteroid insensitivity. *J Allergy Clin Immunol*. 2010;125:550-8.
20. Jonas BS, Wagener DK, Lando JF, Feldman JJ. Symptoms of anxiety and depression as risk factors for development of asthma. *J Appl Biobeh Res*. 1999;4:91-119.
21. Weiser EB. The prevalence of anxiety disorders among adults with asthma: a meta-analytic review. *J Clin Psychol Med Settings*. 2007;14:297-307.

22. Chida Y, Hamer M, Steptoe A. A bidirectional relationship between psychosocial factors and atopic disorders: a systematic review and meta-analysis. *Psychosom Med.* 2008;70: 102-16.

23. Clark DM. A cognitive approach to panic. *Behav Res Ther.* 1986;24:461-70.

24. Dimopoulou T, Pennington D, Wallace L, Bell R, Lawford P, Mansur AH, et al. Clinically anxious asthma patients: the role of catastrophic cognition. *Eur Respir J.* 2006;28:316S.

25. Brown ES, Khan DA, Mahadi S. Psychiatric diagnoses in inner city outpatients with moderate to severe asthma. *Int J Psychiatry Med.* 2000;30:319-27.

26. Solis OL, Khan DA, Brown ES. Age at onset of major depression in inner-city adults with asthma. *Psychosomatics.* 2006;47:330-2.

27. Costello RW, Jacoby DB, Fryer AD. Pulmonary neuronal M2 muscarinic receptor function in asthma and animals models of hyperreactivity. *Thorax.* 1998;53:613-6.

28. Carr RE, Lehrer PM, Hochron SM, Jackson A. Effect of psychological stress on airway impedance in individuals with asthma and panic disorder. *J Abnorm Psychol.* 1996;105: 137-41.

29. Lehrer PM, Hochron S, Carr R, Edelberg R, Hamer R, Jackson A, et al. Behavioural task-induced bronchodilation in asthma during active and passive tasks: a possible cholinergic link to psychologically induced airway changes. *Psychosom Med.* 1996;58:413-22.

30. Miller BD, Wood BL. Influence of specific emotional states on autonomic reactivity and pulmonary function in asthmatic children. *J Am Acad Child Adolesc Psychiatry.* 1997;36:669-77.

31. Katon W, Schulberg H. Epidemiology of depression in primary care. *Gen Hosp Psychiatry.* 1992;14:237-47.

32. Zielinski TA, Brown ES, Nejtek VA, Khan DA, Morre JJ, Rush AJ. Depression in asthma; Prevalence and clinical implications. *Prim Care Companion J Clin Psychiatry.* 2000;2:153-8.

33. Badoux A, Levy DA. Psychologic symptoms in asthma and chronic urticaria. *Ann Allergy.* 1994;72:229-34.

34. Derogatis LR. Brief symptom inventory scale. Hertfordshire: Pearson Education; 2007.

35. Picado C, Montserrat JM, de Pablo J, Plaza V, Agusti-Vidal A. Predisposing factors to death after recovery from a life-threatening asthmatic attack. *J Asthma.* 1989;26:231-6.

36. Allen GM, Hickie I, Gandevia SC, McKenzie DK. Impaired voluntary drive to breathe: a possible link between depression and unexplained ventilatory failure in asthmatic patients. *Thorax.* 1994;49:881-4.

37. Janson S, Reed ML. Patients' perceptions of asthma control and impact on attitudes and self-management. *J Asthma.* 2000;37:625-40.

38. NICE. Management of anxiety (panic disorder with or without agoraphobia and generalised anxiety disorder) in adults in primary, secondary and community care. London; 2004. Available from URL: www.nice.org.uk.

39. Yellowlees PM, Alpers JH, Bowden JJ, Bryant GD, Ruffin RE. Psychiatric morbidity in patients with chronic airflow obstruction. *Med J Aust.* 1987;146:305-7.

40. Yellowlees PM, Kalucy RS. Psychobiological aspects of asthma and the consequent research implications. *Chest.* 1990;97:628-34.

41. Kolbe J, Fergusson W, Vamos M, Garrett J. Case control study of severe life threatening asthma (SLTA) in adults: psychological factors. *Thorax.* 2002;57:317-22.

42. Greaves CJ, Eiser C, Seamark D, Halpin DM. Attack context: an important mediator of the relationship between psychological status and asthma outcomes. *Thorax.* 2002;57: 217-21.

43. Brashear RE. Hyperventilation syndrome. *Lung.* 1983;161:257-73.

44. Christopher KL, Wood RP 2nd, Eckert RC, Blager FB, Raney RA, Souhrada JF. Vocal-cord dysfunction presenting in asthma. *N Engl J Med.* 1983;308:1566-70.

45. Newman KB, Mason UG 3rd, Schmaling KB. Clinical features of vocal cord dysfunction. *Am J Respir Crit Care Med.* 1995;152:1382-6.

46. Van de Van LL, Mouthaan BJ, Hoes MJ. Treatment of hyperventilation syndrome with bisoprolol: a placebo-controlled clinical trial. *J Psychosom Res.* 1995;39:1007-13.

47. Mastrovich JD, Greenberger PA. Psychogenic cough in adults: a report of two cases and review of the literature. *Allergy Asthma Proc.* 2002;23:27-33.

48. Hadan JR, Khan DA. Psychiatric syndromes that mimic asthma. In: Brown ES, editor. Asthma; social and psychological factors and psychosomatic syndromes. New York: Karger; 2003.

49. Bucknall CE, Slack R, Godley CC, Mackay TW, Wright SC. Scottish Confidential Inquiry into Asthma Deaths (SCIAD). *Thorax.* 1999;54:978-84.

50. Burr ML, Davies BH, Hoare A, Jones A, Williamson IJ, Holgate SK, et al. A confidential inquiry into asthma deaths in Wales. *Thorax.* 1999;54:985-9.

51. Mohan G, Harrison BD, Badminton RM, Mildenhall S, Wareham NJ. A confidential enquiry into deaths caused by asthma in an English health region: implications for general practice. *Br J Gen Pract.* 1996;46:529-32.

52. Sturdy PM, Victor CR, Anderson HR, Bland JM, Butland BK, Harrison BD, et al. Mortality and Severe Morbidity Working Group of the National Asthma Task Force. Psychological, social and health behaviour risk factors for deaths certified as asthma: a national case-control study. *Thorax.* 2002;57:1034-9.

53. Miles JF, Garden GM, Tunnicliffe WS, Cayton RM, Ayres JG. Psychological morbidity and coping skills in patients with brittle and non-brittle asthma: a case-control study. *Clin Exp Allergy.* 1997;27:1151-9.

54. Heaney LG, Conway E, Kelly C, Johnston BT, English C, Stevenson M, et al. Predictors of therapy resistant asthma: outcome of a systematic evaluation protocol. *Thorax.* 2003;58:561-6.

55. Heaney LG, Conway E, Kelly C, Gamble J. Prevalence of psychiatric morbidity in a difficult asthma population: relationship to asthma outcome. *Respir Med.* 2005;99:1152-9.

56. Robinson DS, Campbell DA, Durham SR, Pfeffer J, Barnes PJ, Chung KF; Asthma and Allergy Research Group of the National Heart and Lung Institute. Systematic assessment of difficult-to-treat asthma. *Eur Respir J.* 2003;22:478-83.

57. Pooler A. Exacerbations of severe asthma: psychosocial predictors and the impact of a nurse led clinic. 2009 Keele University, UK.

58. Chetta A, Gerra G, Foresi A, Zaimovic A, Del Donno M, Chittolini B, et al. Personality profiles and breathlessness perception in outpatients with different gradings of asthma. *Am J Respir Crit Care Med.* 1998;157:116-22.

59. Boulet LP, Deschesnes F, Turcotte H, Gignac F. Near-fatal asthma: clinical and physio-logic features, perception of bronchoconstriction, and psychologic profile. *J Allergy Clin Immunol.* 1991;88:838-46.

60. ten Brinke A, Ouwerkerk ME, Bel EH, Spinhoven P. Similar psychological characteristics in mild and severe asthma. *J Psychosom Res.* 2001;50:7-10.

61. Kolbe J, Vamos M, Fergusson W, Elkind G, Garrett J. Differential influences on asthma self-management knowledge and self-management behavior in acute severe asthma. *Chest.* 1996;110:1463-8.

62. Vamos M, Kolbe J. Psychological factors in severe chronic asthma. *Aust N Z J Psychiatry.* 1999;33:538-44.

63. Halimi L, Vachier I, Varrin M, Godard P, Pithon G, Chanez P. Interference of psychological factors in difficult-to-control asthma. *Respir Med.* 2007;101:154-61.

64. Kolbe J, Vamos M, Fergusson W, Elkind G. Determinants of management errors in acute severe asthma. *Thorax.* 1998;53:14-20.

65. Lavoie KL, Bouthillier D, Bacon SL, Lemière C, Martin J, Hamid Q, et al. Psychologic distress and maladaptive coping styles in patients with severe vs moderate asthma. *Chest.* 2010;137:1324-31.

66. The Diagnostic and Statistical Manual of Mental Disorders (DSM), *Fourth Edition,* (DSM-IV) 2000.

67. Bernstein JA, Dykewicz MS, Histand P, Patterson R. Potentially fatal asthma and syncope. A new variant of Munchausen's syndrome in sports medicine. *Chest.* 1991;99:763-5.

68. Baker CE, Major E. Munchausen's syndrome. A case presenting as asthma requiring ventilation. *Anaesthesia.* 1994;49:1050-1.

69. Downing ET, Braman SS, Fox MJ, Corrao WM. Factitious asthma. Physiological approach to diagnosis. *JAMA.* 1982;248:2878-81.

70. Heaney LG, Brightling CE, Menzies-Gow A, Stevenson M, Niven RM; British Thoracic Society Difficult Asthma Network. Refractory asthma in the UK: cross-sectional findings from a UK multicentre registry. *Thorax.* 2010;65:787-94.

71. Lewis DA, Smith RE. Steroid-induced psychiatric syndromes. A report of 14 cases and a review of the literature. *J Affect Disord.* 1983;5:319-32.

72. Naber D, Sand P, Heigl B. Psychopathological and neuropsychological effects of 8-days' corticosteroid treatment. A prospective study. *Psychoneuroendocrinology.* 1996;21:25-31.

73. Sirois F. Steroid psychosis: a review. *Gen Hosp Psychiatry.* 2003;25:27-33.

74. Bolanos SH, Khan DA, Hanczyc M, Bauer MS, Dhanani N, Brown ES. Assessment of mood states in patients receiving long-term corticosteroid therapy and in controls with patient-rated and clinician-rated scales. *Ann Allergy Asthma Immunol.* 2004;92:500-5.

75. Brown ES, Chamberlain W, Dhanani N, Paranjpe P, Carmody TJ, Sargeant M. An open-label trial of olanzapine for corticosteroid-induced mood symptoms. *J Affect Disord.* 2004;83:277-81.

76. Wolkowitz OM. Prospective controlled studies of the behavioral and biological effects of exogenous corticosteroids. *Psychoneuroendocrinology.* 1994;19:233-55.

77. Keenan PA, Jacobson MW, Soleymani RM, Mayes MD, Stress ME, Yaldoo DT. The effect on memory of chronic prednisone treatment in patients with systemic disease. *Neurology.* 1996;47:1396-402.

78. NICE. Management of depression in primary and secondary care, London 2004. Available from URL: www.nice.org.uk.

79. Yorke J, Fleming SL, Shuldham C. Psychological interventions for adults with asthma: a systematic review. *Respir Med.* 2007;101:1-14.

80. Smith JR, Mugford M, Holland R, Noble MJ, Harrison BD. Psycho-educational interventions for adults with severe or difficult asthma: a systematic review. *J Asthma.* 2007;44:219-41.

81. Smith JR, Mildenhall S, Noble MJ, Shepstone L, Koutantji M, Mugford M, et al. The Coping with Asthma Study: a randomised controlled trial of a home based, nurse led psychoeducational intervention for adults at risk of adverse asthma outcomes. *Thorax.* 2005;60:1003-11.

82. Brown ES, Vigil L, Khan DA, Liggin JD, Carmody TJ, Rush AJ. A randomized trial of citalopram versus placebo in outpatients with asthma and major depressive disorder: a proof of concept study. *Biol Psychiatry.* 2005;58:865-70.

6 Difficult Asthma in Children

Surendran Thavagnanam, Michael D Shields

INTRODUCTION

Asthma management aims at controlling day-to-day symptoms and preventing acute exacerbations. When asthma is controlled, severe exacerbations should be rare, there should be no more than occasional occurrence of symptoms, no need for rescue medications, and there should be normal exercise tolerance and lung function.[1] Doctors treating children need to balance the aims of asthma management against the potential side effects of the medications necessary to achieve perfect control. Inhaled corticosteroids (ICS) are the most effective controller therapy, and most children can be well controlled with standard and safe doses. However, in some children, ongoing day-to-day symptoms and frequent acute exacerbations occur despite therapy.[2]

Modern asthma guidelines use a stepwise approach to escalating the ICS dose and adding other controller therapies and recommend that before initiating a new drug therapy, doctors should recheck inhaler technique, check adherence to medication, and attempt to eliminate trigger factors,[3,4] as these can influence overall asthma control.[1,3,4]

Difficult asthma in children older than 5 years of age may be defined as poorly controlled asthma with persistent symptoms and/or frequent exacerbations despite treatment with an ICS dosage of at least 800 µg/day (budesonide equivalent) plus a long-acting β_2-agonist (LABA) and/or a leukotriene antagonist (LTA). In children below 5 years of age, a dose of ICS of at least 400 µg/day plus a LTA should have been tried. This therapy should have been assessed over a period of at least 6 months.[1] Difficult asthma also includes children who obtain good symptom control but require a high level of therapy to maintain this state.

Difficult asthma in children is common in primary care and is a common reason for referral to respiratory or allergy services.[5] Although only 5–10% of childhood asthmatics have difficult asthma, they account for a disproportionate share of healthcare costs and often require more than two controller medications, frequent use of oral steroids, and pediatric intensive care unit (PICU) admission.[6] Asthma deaths do not always come from the pool of children who have already been declared as having difficult asthma. Real-life studies of populations show that ICS are underused and often are given intermittently.[7,8] In an analysis of the Saskatchewan Health Database, Canada, which included asthmatic children, Suissa et al. found that even the use of low-dose ICS was associated with a decreased risk of death from asthma.[9] Poor medication adherence is clearly associated with increased asthma exacerbations and risk of dying in children.[9,10]

It is likely that majority of children with apparent difficult asthma do not have true therapy-resistant severe asthma.[11] One study looking at children attending a tertiary center with persistent asthma symptoms despite treatment on Step 4 of the British Thoracic Society (BTS) asthma management guidelines, showed evidence of poor adherence, unsupervised taking of medications in young children, ongoing aeroallergens exposure, and psychosocial problems.[12]

A child is labeled as having true 'therapy-resistant severe asthma', if they continue to have ongoing asthma symptoms despite the physician having dealt satisfactorily with the potentially modifiable issues listed in table 6-1.[13] If the problems (e.g., poor inhaler technique, poor adherence, or ongoing triggers) cannot be overcome, it is not possible to say whether the child has or has not true therapy-resistant severe asthma, but the child certainly may continue to have symptoms and remains with the label 'difficult-to-treat asthma'.

DIFFICULT-TO-TREAT SEVERE ASTHMA

When faced with a child with apparent uncontrolled asthma, considerable time is needed and a systematic approach should be used to address the issues listed in the checklist in table 6-1.

Table 6-1	Checklist of Key Questions and Issues to Address in Children

- What is the basis of asthma diagnosis? Is the asthma diagnosis correct?
- How is the child currently being affected?
- Do the child and family have an asthma management plan that is understood?
- Are the treatments being used appropriately (including use of inhaler device)? Is medication delivery adequate?
- Is the child adhering to the agreed prescribed therapy plan?
- Are there ongoing trigger factors causing further airway inflammation or are there any treatable or avoidable precipitants?
- Is there a concomitant disease that might be affecting asthma or reducing the quality of life in its own right?
- Could the current treatment be making the child worse?
- Are the symptoms being overperceived or being exaggerated?

Is the Asthma Diagnosis Correct?

It is necessary to confirm the diagnosis of asthma in children with difficult-to-treat asthma. This is important but problematic. The recent BTS asthma management guideline acknowledges that there is no defining test for asthma in young children but uses a probability approach (high, intermediate, and low).[1] We find that a good starting point is to summarize the basis upon which the asthma diagnosis was made. An example statement for a classic case of atopic asthma in a young child is given below. The diagnosis of asthma required a clear description of recurrent wheezing that was relieved by antiasthma therapy and was in the setting of atopy.

CASE EXAMPLE DOCUMENTATION ON THE BASIS OF ASTHMA DIAGNOSIS

This 4-year-old girl, who had atopic eczema, also had prolonged episodes of cough and wheezing triggered by head colds (approximately each month). Inbetween, when she was otherwise well, she experienced shortness of breath and wheezing with exercise. The night following a very active day, she coughed throughout the night. There was a strong family history of asthma, eczema and hayfever. Over the last three months with treatment (beclomethasone 200 µg twice daily plus montelukast), she had no further day-to-day exercise or nocturnal symptoms and had only one minor wheezing episode triggered by a head cold.

In preschool children, a 'trial of antiasthma therapy' is often used to support or even confirm an asthma diagnosis. With respect to using such a trial of treatment in clinching an asthma diagnosis, it is important to ensure that a defined objective outcome is recorded, since parents, keen to please the doctor, may report that their child is a little better. It is also important to keep at the back of one's mind that the associated improvement may not have been related to the therapy. This could occur when the treatment trial has been carried out over the spring season, when the child naturally stops experiencing recurrent winter viral infections.

As there is no precise diagnostic test or definition for asthma in early childhood, other conditions may need to be excluded, such as those listed in table 6-2.

Table 6-2	Some Causes of Wheezing in Children
• Non-atopic, recurrent, viral-induced	• Recurrent pulmonary aspiration/gastroesophageal reflux
• Congenital malformation causing airway narrowing	• Tuberculosis
• Cystic fibrosis, primary ciliary dyskinesia, immune deficiency, idiopathic bronchiectasis	• Congenital heart disease
	• Allergic bronchopulmonary aspegillosis
• Retained inhaled foreign body	• Interstitial lung disease

In our experience, there are some scenarios as discussed below that are associated with the 'over-diagnosis' of asthma, and children may end up on unnecessary high doses of antiasthma therapy.

Firstly, the child may not be "wheezy." Young children or toddlers often have noisy breathing due to 'rattles', and this is commonly misunderstood as wheeze. The child is breathing through phlegm that sits in the pharynx or upper trachea and the parents can palpate this chest sound. While for some of these children, this mucous hypersecretion may be the first sign of asthma; for the majority, it simply disappears over time.

Secondly, children may have a chronic productive cough from recurrent infections. Recently, it is increasingly recognized that a number of children are labeled as difficult-to-treat asthmatics, but instead have persistent bacterial bronchitis, which represents a persistent bacterial infection of the conducting airways. These children may be treated with high-dose antiasthma therapy, which is not necessary, as they respond to a prolonged course of antibiotic.[14] The BTS asthma guidelines state that children with isolated cough (no wheeze) have a low probability of asthma.[1]

Thirdly, non-atopic children with episodic viral wheezing have a low probability of asthma and are less likely to respond to regular ICS or even oral steroids during an acute exacerbation.[15,16] Many of these children outgrow wheezing with time, but some can change phenotype and may evolve into a more obvious classical atopic pattern.[17]

Finally, in older children, functional breathing disorders can mimic asthma symptoms and these include:

- Hyperventilation, secondary to anxiety
- Deconditioning, where breathlessness occurs with minimal exercise due to physiological limitation rather than exercise-induced asthma. This is commonly associated with obesity
- Vocal cord dysfunction (VCD), which is an upper airway obstruction caused by paradoxical adduction of the vocal cords on inspiration. It is more common in older girls and often misdiagnosed as asthma. VCD is diagnosed by laryngoscopy, and in one study of severe asthma in children, 14% of the children had VCD.[18] During an acute severe episode, patients with VCD may show flattening of the inspiratory portion of the flow-volume loop, and they usually have a normal chest X-ray (CXR) and normal arterial CO_2 and O_2.

It is important to remember that functional breathing disorders can occur in children with asthma and may make asthma symptoms appear severe. This makes it hard to be certain of the relative contributions of both conditions on the reported symptoms.

Rarely, a child may be seen with wheezing and fixed airways obstruction following a respiratory tract infection (e.g., adenovirus) or Stevens-Johnson syndrome and has bronchiolitis obliterans or constrictive bronchiolitis. This diagnosis has traditionally required a lung biopsy to show narrowing and/or complete obliteration of the small airways. More recently, it has been shown that open lung biopsy can be avoided in some children with a characteristic computed tomography (CT) scan, which includes parenchymal hypoattenuation, vascular attenuation, and bronchial narrowing.[19] However, another study reported considerable overlap in CT scans between those with severe asthma and bronchiolitis obliterans.[20] Children with wheezing and obstructive spirometry should have an assessment of their bronchodilator responsiveness (BDR) made. BDR may need to be checked after a course of oral steroids before fixed airway obstruction can be confirmed.

Do the Child and Parents Understand the Written Asthma Management Plan?

Modern asthma management guidelines stress the fundamental importance that children and parents should have an individualized written asthma management plan that they can understand and follow.[1] Parents need to know what each medication does, and when it should be used. It would be unnatural for a parent to be expected to give their well child regular controller ICS, if the preventative properties have not been explained.

Is the Medication Being Delivered?

Ensuring that children can effectively take inhalers and deliver medication into their lungs is part of usual asthma practice but needs to be checked frequently. Adequately delivering inhaled medications to young children can be problematic with child cooperation being the major limiting factor. Crying and struggling during treatment with inhalers or trying to administer inhaled therapy while a child is asleep is associated with delivery of almost no medication.[21,22] If this intolerance of ICS therapy (inhaler/face mask or nebulized) cannot be overcome, second best prevention therapy that can be used, is oral montelukast or theophylline.[1] Some of these children may become well controlled, but many remain as difficult-to-treat asthmatics.

Is the Child Adhering to Therapy?

It is a common misconception to think that parents with a child with severe asthma symptoms will be more diligent and conscientious.[23] Poor adherence to therapy is a major cause of difficult-to-treat asthma.[12]

Whether it is intentional (e.g., parent has concerns about the side effects of steroids and, therefore, never collect the inhaler) or unintentional (forgetting, most likely due to a chaotic household), non-adherence is difficult to detect.[24] Direct questioning is unreliable in children.[10] An accurate method involves using an electronic logger to time and date each actuation. These devices are helpful to define the extent of the problem, but they are not currently feasible in everyday practice. The majority of general practitioners in UK have electronic prescribing, and it is possible to obtain a review of the previous 3, 6, or 12 months of prescription refills requested and collected and to calculate the average daily ICS inhalations. The use of repeat prescription records improves non-adherence detection compared to detailed parental questioning; however, it is still not as accurate as use of the electronic data logger.[10] Recent evidence suggests that if doctors are prepared to obtain the electronic prescription records before the consultation and to use it in a non-confrontational 'concordance feedback interview' then adherence behavior can be modified.[25,26] Additionally, adherence can also be inferred from blood levels measured from children on theophylline or oral prednisolone. In the future, affordable inhalers may become available that provide adherence feedback to both the child and the physician, and research is ongoing to see if they can ultimately improve asthma control. Because it is so difficult to truly confirm therapy adherence in children, it is worth considering observing the effects of giving a long-acting depot systemic steroid, e.g., triamcinolone,[27] which when given intramuscularly will demonstrate true steroid responsiveness. Depot intramuscular injections of triamcinolone carry a risk of subcutaneous atrophy at the injection site, which would accumulate if repeated monthly injections were used. An alternative strategy would be to arrange for a period of directly observed delivery of asthma therapy by an asthma nurse or trained school teacher.

Are there Ongoing Triggers Factors?

Triggering factors that are associated with asthma include:

- *Environmental tobacco smoke (ETS) exposure:* Exposure to cigarette smoke is a direct airway irritant and in adults, smoking creates a state of relative ICS resistance. Passive smoking is common in children with asthma, including those with difficult-to-treat asthma. Cigarette exposure in the home or car is associated with severe asthma and pediatric intensive care admission.[28-31]
- *Dampness, indoor mold, and continuing allergen exposure:* Exposure to indoor mold has been consistently associated with adverse respiratory health outcomes in children.[32] However, the beneficial effect of improved home heating and ventilation systems has not been consistent.[33,34] Although there is a debate as to whether early exposure to aeroallergens in infancy is helpful for prevention of asthma, reducing exposure to aeroallergens to which children with asthma are sensitized, or on which triggers asthma attacks seems to be logical.[35-37] Ongoing exposure of the airway epithelium to aeroallergens in sensitized children is likely to maintain airway inflammation. However, there is limited evidence for benefit, perhaps, because many of our interventions do little to reduce the allergen load. Glasgow et al. reported no difference in respiratory symptoms,

one year after house dust mite-occlusive mattress covers were introduced in mite sensitive moderate-to-severe asthmatic children.[35] It is important to remember that children spend a considerable amount of time in school classrooms, which may also be damp, cold, moldy, and have aeroallergens.

Is there a Concomitant Disease that might Be Affecting Asthma or Reducing the Quality of Life in Its Own Right?

Allergic Rhinitis and Rhinosinusitis

Allergic rhinitis (AR) causes a significant reduction in children's quality of life and should be treated in its own right.[38,39] AR often coexists with atopic asthma and is associated with more severe asthma and hospital admissions.[40] AR therefore should not go unrecognized and untreated. However, there is little evidence that specific AR treatment results in improvement in asthma.[41] Both symptomatic and asymptomatic rhinosinusitis have been reported to occur more frequently in children with severe asthma and, therefore, may require formal ear, nose, and throat (ENT) assessment and treatment.[42]

Obesity and Obstructive Sleep Apnea

Recent studies have reported a higher incidence of asthma in obese children. Young obese children have twice the odds of having asthma compared to children with normal weight.[43] However, the evidence that obesity is associated with more severe asthma is limited.[44,45] From an epidemiological view, country per capita sugar consumption is associated with more severe childhood asthma.[44] In the Childhood Asthma Management Program (CAMP) study, overweight or obese children showed a reduced response to ICS and increased emergency room (EM) visits.[46] A high fat diet impairs bronchodilator responses and is associated with increased neutrophilic airway inflammation in asthmatics.[47] Tackling obesity is difficult but worth trying, as it could have other long-term health benefits for the child. However, it is unknown if weight loss will cause asthma improvement.[47] With respect to the obese child with respiratory symptoms, it is important to confirm that the symptoms are due to asthma and not shortness of breath on exercise due to deconditioning. In a group of children with difficult-to-treat asthma, 36% of whom were obese, the prevalence of obstructive sleep apnea was high and treatment with adenotonsillectomy was associated with improvements in asthma severity.[48]

Psychological and Mental Health Issues

A recent review of the literature concluded that behavioral problems and a lower quality of life are pronounced in children and adolescents with difficult-to-treat asthma. This suggests that healthcare professionals should assess and, if necessary, treat behavioral problems.[49] However, although recommended, there is no strong evidence that family therapy improves asthma control.[49,50] Depression or stress in children with asthma may go unrecognized and untreated. The impact of treating comorbid mental health issues in asthmatic children is unknown but is worth pursuing.

Could the Current Treatment Be Making the Child Worse?

When children are inadequately controlled with ICS, the BTS asthma guidelines recommend sequential trials of LABA, LTA, increasing ICS dosage, and theophylline. This approach has been confirmed in a recent "step-up study" which suggested that an individual child has a differential response to (i) doubling ICS, (ii) adding LABA, or (iii) adding LTA.[51]

The addition of LABA to ICS is beneficial in children for at least up to 3 months duration in terms of improving symptom control and reduced exacerbations. Bisgaard et al. first highlighted the potential of LABA therapy to be associated with more severe exacerbations.[52] Weinberger et al. reported cases of two boys who stopped having acute exercise-induced asphyxia asthma attacks when LABA were stopped.[53] Furthermore, the effect on exercise of regular use of LABA wanes over time even when ICS are used.[54,55] Despite the recent FDA black box warning on the use of LABA in children, the true existence or explanation for this paradox (where the addition of LABA improves overall asthma control but might be rarely associated with severe exacerbations) is unclear. It is also unclear, but unlikely, that taking into account an individual's genotype will be helpful.[51] With this in mind, it would be wise to consider the possibility that an individual child could experience better asthma control, if a different second line therapy to a LABA was tried. When using a LABA the combination inhalers (ICS plus LABA) are recommended as they prevent the possibility for differential adherence where only the LABA can be used.

Are the Symptoms Being Overperceived or Being Exaggerated?

Although there is little objective literature regarding children's perceptions of airway obstruction and the use of inhaled bronchodilators, we have seen children who feel the need to take their reliever inhaler several times during a clinic consultation, because they felt 'tight' but yet had an entirely normal chest examination and normal lung function at that time. In addition, the authors have seen children whose asthma has only come under control after a legal dispute has been resolved to the parent's satisfaction. On the other hand, the inability to perceive the severity of asthma symptoms is a risk factor for near-fatal asthma.[56]

INVESTIGATION AND FILTERING OF CASES OF DIFFICULT-TO-TREAT ASTHMA

In a cohort of well characterized children with apparent difficult asthma, Konradasen et al. found that 39% had potentially modifiable or treatable factors.[57]

These exacerbating factors have not been disclosed during routine care but only became apparent after applying an extensive standardized clinical protocol. As a result of this study, children with difficult-to-treat asthma (but not necessarily therapy-resistant severe asthma) were identified. Factors associated with DTA included lower socioeconomic class and an elevated fractional exhaled nitric oxide (FeNO) level. However, the commonly used cutoff point for the childhood-asthma control test seemed to underestimate the number of children with uncontrolled asthma.[57] Clearly, many children with difficult-to-treat asthma have factors that should be modifiable and which, when addressed, could bring their asthma to satisfactory control.

Apart from teenagers with compliance issues, most children are not in a position to take adequate action to address the points mentioned. They cannot stop their parents smoking and nor can get their parents to collect prescription refills, even if they would be enthusiastic therapy adherers. Many asthma clinics in both primary care and hospital are not set up to do a detailed assessment of adherence. Doctors may not take the time to find out about a child's repeat prescription record and may not feel comfortable to use the information by giving feedback.

It is important to determine, if there are other comorbidities, which are contributing to the child's overall poor asthma control, and further investigations should be performed to rule out other possibilities of alternate diagnoses. Suggested investigations include esophageal monitoring to rule out gastroesophageal reflux disease (GERD); sweat test to rule out cystic fibrosis; nasal brush biopsy, and/or nasal nitric oxide to rule out primary ciliary dyskinesia; serum IgA, IgM, IgG, and specific antibody response to vaccination to rule out underlying immunodeficiency.

Bush et al. recently stressed the importance of providing a program of intensive investigation to filter out difficult-to-treat asthmatics from those children with true therapy-resistant severe asthma.[58] They suggest that an initial hospital-based assessment (Table 6-3) followed by a home visit (Table 6-4) could identify potentially modifiable factors in more than 50% of cases.[58]

Once convinced that the child has true therapy-resistant asthma and that the modifiable factors have been addressed, Bush et al. suggests more invasive investigations using the second of a two stage approach.[58] The aim of this is to find out if there is an additional as yet undiscovered diagnosis, to determine the extent and type of airway inflammation and whether there is any response to an intramuscular (IM) injection of depot triamcinolone. In this second stage assessment, the children have (i) symptom and bronchodilator use evaluation, (ii) spirometry and bronchodilator responsiveness, (iii) FeNO and induced sputum repeated. This is followed by more invasive tests to include a bronchoscopy with bronchoalveolar lavage and endobronchial biopsy and 24-hour pH studies. The noninvasive tests are repeated one month after a single IM injection of triamcinolone.

Table 6-3	Tests at Hospital Visit

1. Allergy tests:
   a. Skin prick tests to aeroallergens (grass and tree pollen, cat and dog, cockroach and house dust mite), food allergens (milk, egg, peanut), and fungi (including *Aspergillus fumigatus* and *Alternaria alternate*)
   b. Total and specific IgE testing
2. Fractional exhaled nitric oxide (FeNO), which is a noninvasive assessment of allergy airways inflammation
3. Spirometry and bronchodilator responsiveness
4. Induced sputum (only if $FEV_1 > 70\%$) for differential cell count or cough swab to identify persistent bacterial endobronchial infection and presences of *Aspergillus*, which may contribute to the diagnosis of allergic bronchopulmonary aspergillosis
5. Saliva cotinine – an objective measure of environmental tobacco smoke (ETS) exposure
6. Drug-blood concentrations, e.g., theophylline or prednisolone assay
7. Consideration of need for an HRCT to determine the presence of bronchiectasis or bronchiolitis obliterans

Table 6-4	Areas to Be Assessed by Home Visit Nurse

The home visit by a well-trained nurse is used to assess the following four areas:

1. Adherence; family is asked to produce medication – with a check made on expiry date, drug delivery device/inhaler technique, prescription refills collected
2. Exposure to environmental tobacco smoke (e.g., ETS)
3. Ongoing allergen exposure
4. Psychosocial issues

Table 6-5	Severe Asthma Clinical Phenotypes

The severe asthma clinical phenotypes include a spectrum of illnesses that are as follows:

1. Episodic obstruction: Episodic severe exacerbations with normal intercurrent lung function and relatively mild intercurrent symptoms
2. Persistent symptoms: Day-to-day symptoms but with relatively normal lung function (other than during an exacerbation)
3. Persistent obstruction: Severe persistent asthma with debilitating day-to-day symptoms and persistent reduced lung function, interspersed with exacerbations

THERAPY-RESISTANT SEVERE ASTHMA

There appears to be a spectrum with at least two different clinical phenotypes of children with severe asthma (Table 6-5). At one extreme are children who are prone to having severe exacerbations but who have relatively few symptoms and normal lung function inbetween exacerbations. The exacerbations may be frequent or infrequent, and while all children can suffer severe exacerbations, some come on gradually over 12–24 hours, e.g., triggered by a an upper respiratory tract infection (URTI), while others are more 'brittle' with almost an anaphylactic onset. On the other hand, there are a group of children with chronic persistent day-to-day symptoms. Children with severe persistent symptoms are more likely to have reduced lung function, bronchial hyper-reactivity, increased serum total IgE, and sensitivity to multiple allergens.[59]

Pathology

Children who have died from acute asthma have severe airway mucous obstruction and marked smooth muscle hypertrophy. Like adults, children with severe asthma have reticular basement membrane thickening,[60,61] although this alone is unlikely to contribute much to the airways obstruction. Jenkins et al. reported that FEV_1 was not related to the basement membrane thickness in six children with severe asthma.[62] Regamy et al.[63] demonstrated the increased airway smooth muscle mass and Barbato et al.[64] reported evidence for increased in angiogenesis in children with severe asthma. Most interestingly, in children (5–15 years) with severe asthma, Tillie-Leblond et al. reported that the reticular basement membrane was equally thickened in those with episodic obstruction and those with persistent airways obstruction. However, reduced FEV_1 in children with persistent airway obstruction was related to increased surface area of airway smooth muscle and increased number of blood vessels.[65]

Risk Factors for Near-fatal or Fatal Asthma Attacks

Children with severe life threatening asthma attacks may be from either difficult-to-treat asthma or true severe asthma groupings and consistent risk factors include previous severe exacerbations in the last year (PICU admission, >2 hospitalizations, and >3 emergency department attendances), obesity, low socioeconomic family, very frequent use of β_2-agonist, and the inability to perceive the severity of their asthma symptoms.

Phenotype Targeting of Therapy

There has been a great deal of interest in the inflammatory cell phenotype of children with severe asthma. Children with mild-to-moderate atopic asthma typically have elevated eosinophils in bronchoalveolar lavage fluid.[66] This may be relevant to treatments since eosinophilic inflammation in asthma is considered more likely steroid responsive. Predominantly neutrophilic airway inflammation may be associated with steroid use, which has been associated with prolonging neutrophil survival. Alternatively, neutrophilic inflammation may be due to the persistence of microbial infection in the airway. *Mycoplasma*, *Chlamydia*, bacteria, and viruses have variably been associated with severe asthma.[67] Paucicellular airway inflammation may be the result of effective anti-inflammatory steroid therapy.[62]

Bush et al. suggested an approach that used the type of airway inflammation (eosinophilic vs. neutrophilic) to partially direct therapy in children with true therapy-resistant severe asthma.[58] For those with eosinophilic airway inflammation, they suggest using a higher dose ICS or the single maintenance and reliever therapy (SMART) approach, where the combined budesonide/formoterol inhaler is used as both maintenance and reliever therapy. This results in the child receiving a much higher dose of ICS at the start of an exacerbation along with a fast but long-acting bronchodilator. This approach has been associated with fewer exacerbations.[52,68] If higher dose ICS therapy is not effective, they recommend systemic (IM) triamcinolone. This approach not only overcomes the ever present problem of poor adherence but will help determine, if the child's asthma is truly steroid resistant. Anti-IgE therapy with omalizumab is next recommended for children whose IgE is elevated, but less than 1500 IU/mL.

For predominantly neutrophilic airway inflammation, they suggest using theophyllines and macrolide antibiotics.

Paucicellular inflammation, as determined using induced sputum in severe asthma, has been described to be relatively common.[69] Bush et al. suggest that, in this situation, steroids should be reduced.[58] However, Jenkins et al. in their case series noted little in the way of airway inflammation, but with continued use of high-dose systemic steroids, were able to provide further worthwhile improvement in lung function.[62]

Although logical, there is little evidence to suggest that a specific inflammation phenotype approach to therapy is beneficial in improving control for true severe asthma.

OVERVIEW OF AVAILABLE TREATMENTS FOR THERAPY-RESISTANT SEVERE ASTHMA

Children with severe asthma have traditionally been treated with regular systemic steroids and to accept the side effects that occur. They typically reach this position when frequent bursts of systemic steroids merge into continuous treatment. Children, especially teenagers, do not like the side effects of steroids on body image, and systemic steroids are well known to carry long-term risks to health, adversely affecting bone metabolism, linear growth, and adrenal function.

In this section, we summarize potential therapies that can be used to prevent a child requiring regular oral steroids in the first place (moving from BTS asthma management guideline steps 4 and 5) or which could help provide added benefits to asthma, still uncontrolled by oral steroids (BTS asthma guideline step 5). Apart from the use of anti-IgE therapy, the quality of evidence is limited.

Very High-dose Inhaled Corticosteroids

For majority of children with mild-to-moderate severe asthma, there appears to be a dose response plateau with little extra benefit gained from using higher doses,[70] but there are no randomized controlled trials (RCTs) using very high doses ICS (>800 μg BD equivalent per day). While by no means completely safe, it seems logical and potentially safer to give a trial of higher dose ICS (>800 μg/day budesonide equivalent) prior to placing a child on to regular long-term oral steroids. Like children treated with long-term systemic steroids, those on very high-dose of ICS should be assumed to have a degree of adrenal gland suppression. Therapy should not be stopped suddenly and consideration should be given to short-term steroid cover for significant febrile illness or surgery.

Fine Particle Inhaled Corticosteroids

Distal small airway and alveolar allergic inflammation may still persist in asthmatics despite using the conventional ICS.[71] The newer chlorofluorocarbon (CFC) free ICS (BDP-HFA, QVAR® and ciclesonide) have steroid molecules of a finer particle size, which therefore, can penetrate further down the bronchial tree providing better anti-inflammatory effect to the small airways. A small case series of children with severe asthma suggested that replacing fluticasone with the particle ICS (ciclesonide) maintained similar asthma control but allowed the adrenal suppression to recover.[72]

Macrolide Antibiotics

Macrolide antibiotics may have an immunomodulatory effect and reduce both neutrophilic inflammation and drive type 2 helper T lymphocytes (Th2) toward a non-allergic Th1 phenotype.[73] In addition, they may have an antimicrobial action against both typical and atypical organisms that have been detected in the lower airways of asthmatics. Despite positive case reports, this therapy has not been adequately studied. However, an underpowered RCT in children with apparent severe asthma did not suggest a huge benefit when azithromycin was added to ICS plus LABA or when compared with the addition of montelukast.[11]

Anti-IgE Therapy

Omalizumab is a humanized monoclonal anti-IgE used for the treatment of severe allergic asthma and is licensed for use in children aged 6 years and above whose IgE is elevated but less than 1500 IU/mL. It has a low frequency of side effects (apart from a local injection site irritation). Compared to placebo, older children and adults treated with omalizumab were more likely to be able to completely withdraw from oral steroids and had reduced risk of exacerbations.[74] Omalizumab as add-on therapy to ICS has been studied in children, 6–12 years of age with moderate-to-severe asthma and has been shown to reduce significant clinical exacerbations over a period of 52 weeks. The majority of children were taking ICS with both a LABA and LTA. A recent study showed that when added to guidelines-based therapy, omalizumab further improved asthma control, nearly eliminated seasonal peaks in exacerbations, and reduced the need for other medications to control asthma.[75]

Terbutaline Infusion

Continuous subcutaneous infusion of terbutaline has been reported to be beneficial in children with severe asthma. Payne et al. reported that five of eight children experienced a symptomatic improvement additional to treatment with regular oral prednisolone.[76] The efficacy and safety of this therapy has not been assessed in a RCT. It is the authors experience and impression that this form of treatment initially works well, but the beneficial effects wane over time.

Immunotherapy

A recent RCT of house dust mite (HDM)-specific immunotherapy in children with moderate-to-severe asthma reported benefit, including reduced emergency room visits and admissions.[77] However another study of children whose asthma was controlled with adequate pharmacotherapy and HDM avoidance measures, the addition of HDM sublingual immunotherapy did not provide additional benefit compared with placebo, despite a significant reduction in allergic response to HDM.[78] The role of specific immunotherapy remains unclear in children with severe asthma.[16]

Other Treatments for True Steroid Resistant Severe Childhood Asthma

The BTS asthma management guideline has included immunosuppressants, such as methotrexate, ciclosporin, intravenous gammaglobulin, and oral gold, as possible antiasthma therapies that may allow a decrease in the long-term steroid requirements. These therapies have significant side effects and their effectiveness in childhood asthma is unknown.

Our experience with the very occasional use of intravenous gammaglobulin or methotrexate to treat therapy resistant asthma has been extremely disappointing. The addition of low-dose ciclosporin has been reported in a small case series to allow steroid reduction in some children.[79]

INTERMITTENT EPISODIC SEVERE VIRAL-TRIGGERED ASTHMA

Until recently, asthma management guidelines have assumed that children with intermittent symptoms have mild asthma. Clearly, there are a group of children with intermittent asthma who are not mild but experience severe life-threatening attacks. Significant coughing and upper respiratory signs often precede severe wheezing episodes.[80] Current evidence suggests that young preschool children with episodic viral-triggered wheezing do not respond well to regular ICS.[15,16] If these children do not have any evidence of ongoing airway inflammation in the interval periods between viral exacerbations, it is possible that the regular use of high doses of ICS will be associated with the potential for greater side effects (better absorption of ICS from noninflamed airways). In addition, in young children, oral steroids even when initiated by parents early in the illness may not work well.[81] Parent-initiated prednisolone has a small beneficial effect when given to school-age children at the start of an acute asthma exacerbation.[82] There is evidence that intermittent use of high-dose ICS (nebulized budesonide) or intermittent use of montelukast may have a small beneficial effect on the severity of the exacerbation.[83]

Despite the lack of good evidence, we aim to treat such difficult to manage children with severe intermittent viral-induced wheezing with a low background dose of ICS when well. In the written action plan, the parents are told to (i) increase the dose of ICS (usually by switching to nebulized budesonide 1–2 mg 2–4 times/day and (ii) to start oral montelukast at the first sign of a head cold. Once wheezing starts, bronchodilators and oral steroids are commenced and parents are advised to seek help early, if wheezing becomes more severe.

REFERENCES

1. British Thoracic Society Scottish Intercollegiate Guidelines Network. British Guideline on the Management of Asthma. *Thorax*. 2008;63:iv1-121.
2. Rabe KF, Adachi M, Lai CK, Soriano JB, Vermeire PA, Weiss KB, et al. Worldwide severity and control of asthma in children and adults: the global asthma insights and reality surveys. *J Allergy Clin Immunol*. 2004;114:40-7.
3. FitzGerald M, Barnes PJ, Barnes N, Bateman ED, Becker A, Drazen JM, et al. Global Strategy for Asthma Management and Prevention, Global Initiative for Asthma (GINA) 2010. Available from URL: http://www.ginasthma.org. Accessed June/30, 2010.
4. Expert Panel Report 3: Guidelines for the Diagnosis and Management of Asthma, Full Report 2007. Available from URL: http://www.nhlbi.nih.gov/guidelines/asthma/asthgdln.htm.
5. Thomas M, Murray-Thomas T, Fan T, Williams T, Taylor S. Prescribing patterns of asthma controller therapy for children in UK primary care: a cross-sectional observational study. *BMC Pulm Med*. 2010;10-29.
6. Chipps BE, Szefler SJ, Simons FE, Haselkorn T, Mink DR, Deniz Y, et al. Demographic and clinical characteristics of children and adolescents with severe or difficult-to-treat asthma. *J Allergy Clin Immunol*. 2007;119:1156-63.
7. Blais L, Kettani FZ, Lemiere C, Beauchesne MF, Perreault S, Elftouh N, et al. Inhaled corticosteroids vs. leukotriene-receptor antagonists and asthma exacerbations in children. *Respir Med*. 2011;105:846-55.
8. Pando S, Lemière C, Beauchesne MF, Perreault S, Forget A, Blais L. Suboptimal use of inhaled corticosteroids in children with persistent asthma: inadequate prescription, poor drug adherence, or both? *Pharmacotherapy*. 2010;30:1109-16.
9. Suissa S, Ernst P, Kezouh A. Regular use of inhaled corticosteroids and the long term prevention of hospitalisation for asthma. *Thorax*. 2002;57:880-4.

10. Bender B, Wamboldt FS, O'Connor SL, Rand C, Szefler S, Milgrom H, et al. Measurement of children's asthma medication adherence by self report, mother report, canister weight, and Doser CT. *Ann Allergy Asthma Immunol.* 2000;85:416-21.

11. Strunk RC, Bacharier LB, Phillips BR, Szefler SJ, Zeiger RS, Chinchilli VM, et al. Azithromycin or montelukast as inhaled corticosteroid-sparing agents in moderate-tosevere childhood asthma study. *J Allergy Clin Immunol.* 2008;122:1138-44.e4.

12. Bracken M, Fleming L, Hall P, Van Stiphout N, Bossley C, Biggart E, et al. The importance of nurse-led home visits in the assessment of children with problematic asthma. *Arch Dis Child.* 2009;94:780-4.

13. Bush A, Zar HJ. WHO universal definition of severe asthma. *Curr Opin Allergy Clin Immunol.* 2011;11:115-21.

14. Chang AB, Redding GJ, Everard ML. Chronic wet cough: protracted bronchitis, chronic suppurative lung disease and bronchiectasis. *Pediatr Pulmonol.* 2008;43:519-31.

15. McKean M, Ducharme F. Inhaled steroids for episodic viral wheeze of childhood. *Cochrane Database Syst Rev.* 2000;2:CD001107.

16. Grigg J. Role of systemic steroids in acute preschool wheeze. *Arch Dis Child.* 2010;95:491-2.

17. Schultz A, Devadason SG, Savenije OE, Sly PD, Le Souëf PN, Brand PL. The transient value of classifying preschool wheeze into episodic viral wheeze and multiple trigger wheeze. *Acta Paediatr.* 2010;99:56-60.

18. Hicks M, Brugman SM, Katial R. Vocal cord dysfunction/paradoxical vocal fold motion. *Prim Care.* 2008;35:81-103, vii.

19. Smith KJ, Dishop MK, Fan LL, Moonnumakal SP, Smith EO'Brain, Bayindir P, et al. Diagnosis of bronchiolitis obliterans with computed tomography in children. *Pediatr Allergy, Immunol, Pulmonol.* 2010;23:253-9.

20. Bandeira T, Negreiro F, Ferreira R, Salgueiro M, Lobo L, Aguiar P, et al. Clinical, radiological, and physiological differences between obliterative bronchiolitis and problematic severe asthma in adolescents and young adults: the early origins of the overlap syndrome? *Pediatr Pulmonol.* 2011;46:573-80.

21. Marguet C, Couderc L, Le Roux P, Jeannot E, Lefay V, Mallet E. Inhalation treatment: errors in application and difficulties in acceptance of the devices are frequent in wheezy infants and young children. *Pediatr Allergy Immunol.* 2001;12:224-30.

22. Esposito-Festen J, Ijsselstijn H, Hop W, van Vliet F, de Jongste J, Tiddens H. Aerosol therapy by pressured metered-dose inhaler-spacer in sleeping young children: to do or not to do? *Chest.* 2006;130:487-92.

23. Gustafsson PM, Watson L, Davis KJ, Rabe KF. Poor asthma control in children: evidence from epidemiological surveys and implications for clinical practice. *Int J Clin Pract.* 2006;60:321-34.

24. Koster ES, Wijga AH, Koppelman GH, Postma DS, Brunekreef B, De Jongste JC, et al. Uncontrolled asthma at age 8: the importance of parental perception towards medication. *Pediatr Allergy Immunol.* 2011;22:462-8.

25. Williams LK, Peterson EL, Wells K, Campbell J, Wang M, Chowdhry VK, et al. A cluster-randomized trial to provide clinicians inhaled corticosteroid adherence information for their patients with asthma. *J Allergy Clin Immunol.* 2010;126:225-31, 231.e1-4.

26. Weinstein AG. Should patients with persistent severe asthma be monitored for medication adherence? *Ann Allergy Asthma Immunol.* 2005;94:251-7.

27. Panickar JR, Bhatnagar N, Grigg J. Exhaled nitric oxide after a single dose of intramuscular triamcinolone in children with difficult to control asthma. *Pediatr Pulmonol.* 2007; 42:573-8.

28. Mannino DM, Homa DM, Redd SC. Involuntary smoking and asthma severity in children: data from the Third National Health and Nutrition Examination Survey. *Chest.* 2002;122:409-15.

29. Weitzman M, Gortmaker S, Walker DK, Sobol A. Maternal smoking and childhood asthma. *Pediatrics.* 1990;85:505-11.

30. Samir S, Colin Y, Thomas S. Impact of environmental tobacco smoke on children admitted with status asthmaticus in the pediatric intensive care unit. *Pediatr Pulmonol.* 2010.

31. Halterman JS, Fagnano M, Conn KM, Szilagyi PG. Do parents of urban children with persistent asthma ban smoking in their homes and cars? *Ambul Pediatr.* 2006;6:115-9.

32. Antova T, Pattenden S, Brunekreef B, Heinrich J, Rudnai P, Forastiere F, et al. Exposure to indoor mould and children's respiratory health in the PATY study. *J Epidemiol Community Health.* 2008;62:708-14.

33. Wright GR, Howieson S, McSharry C, McMahon AD, Chaudhuri R, Thompson J, et al. Effect of improved home ventilation on asthma control and house dust mite allergen levels. *Allergy.* 2009;64:1671-80.

34. Howden-Chapman P, Pierse N, Nicholls S, Gillespie-Bennett J, Viggers H, Cunningham M, et al. Effects of improved home heating on asthma in community dwelling children: randomised controlled trial. *BMJ.* 2008;337:a1411.

35. Glasgow NJ, Ponsonby AL, Kemp A, Tovey E, van Asperen P, McKay K, et al. Feather bedding and childhood asthma associated with house dust mite sensitisation: a randomised controlled trial. *Arch Dis Child.* 2011;96:541-7.

36. Roy A, Downes MJ, Wisnivesky JP. Comprehensive environmental management of asthma and pediatric preventive care. *Pediatr Allergy Immunol.* 2011;22:277-82.

37. Ahluwalia SK, Matsui EC. The indoor environment and its effects on childhood asthma. *Curr Opin Allergy Clin Immunol.* 2011;11:137-43.

38. Brozek JL, Bousquet J, Baena-Cagnani CE, Bonini S, Canonica GW, Casale TB, et al. Allergic Rhinitis and its Impact on Asthma (ARIA) guidelines: 2010 revision. *J Allergy Clin Immunol.* 2010;126:466-76.

39. Kang HY, Park CS, Bang HR, Sazonov V, Kim CJ. Effect of allergic rhinitis on the use and cost of health services by children with asthma. *Yonsei Med J.* 2008;49:521-9.

40. de Groot EP, Duiverman EJ, Brand PL. Comorbidities of asthma during childhood: possibly important, yet poorly studied. *Eur Respir J.* 2010;36:671-8.

41. Pedroletti C, Lundahl J, Alving K, Hedlin G. Effect of nasal steroid treatment on airway inflammation determined by exhaled nitric oxide in allergic schoolchildren with perennial rhinitis and asthma. *Pediatr Allergy Immunol.* 2008;19:219-26.

42. Pawankar R, Zernotti ME. Rhinosinusitis in children and asthma severity. *Curr Opin Allergy Clin Immunol.* 2009;9:151-3.

43. Suglia SF, Chambers EC, Rosario A, Duarte CS. Asthma and obesity in three-year-old urban children: role of sex and home environment. *J Pediatr.* 2011;159:14-20.e1.

44. Thornley S, Stewart A, Marshall R, Jackson R. Per capita sugar consumption is associated with severe childhood asthma: an ecological study of 53 countries. *Prim Care Respir J.* 2011;20:75-8.

45. Peters JI, McKinney JM, Smith B, Wood P, Forkner E, Galbreath AD. Impact of obesity in asthma: evidence from a large prospective disease management study. *Ann Allergy Asthma Immunol.* 2011;106:30-5.

46. Forno E, Lescher R, Strunk R, Weiss S, Fuhlbrigge A, Celedón JC, et al. Decreased response to inhaled steroids in overweight and obese asthmatic children. *J Allergy Clin Immunol.* 2011;127:741-9.

47. Wood LG, Garg ML, Gibson PG. A high-fat challenge increases airway inflammation and impairs bronchodilator recovery in asthma. *J Allergy Clin Immunol.* 2011;127:1133-40.

48. McCurdy LE, Winterbottom KE, Mehta SS, Roberts JR. Using nature and outdoor activity to improve children's health. *Curr Probl Pediatr Adolesc Health Care.* 2010;40:102-17.

49. Kheirandish-Gozal L, Dayyat EA, Eid NS, Morton RL, Gozal D. Obstructive sleep apnea in poorly controlled asthmatic children: effect of adenotonsillectomy. *Pediatr Pulmonol.* 2011;46:913-8.

50. Verkleij M, van de Griendt EJ, Kaptein AA, van Essen-Zandvliet L, Duiverman E, Geenen R. Behavioral problems in children and adolescents with difficult-to-treat asthma. *J Asthma.* 2011;48:18-24.

51. Lemanske RF Jr, Mauger DT, Sorkness CA, Jackson DJ, Boehmer SJ, Martinez FD, et al. Step-up therapy for children with uncontrolled asthma receiving inhaled corticosteroids. *N Engl J Med.* 2010;362:975-85.

52. Bisgaard H, Le Roux P, Bjåmer D, Dymek A, Vermeulen JH, Hultquist C. Budesonide/formoterol maintenance plus reliever therapy: a new strategy in pediatric asthma. *Chest.* 2006;130:1733-43.

53. Weinberger M, Abu-Hasan M. Life-threatening asthma during treatment with salmeterol. *N Engl J Med.* 2006;355:852-3.

54. Grzelewski T, Stelmach I. Exercise-induced bronchoconstriction in asthmatic children: a comparative systematic review of the available treatment options. *Drugs.* 2009;69:1533-53.

55. Carroll WD, Jones PW, Boit P, Clayton S, Cliff I, Lenney W. Childhood evaluation of salmeterol tolerance—a double-blind randomized controlled trial. *Pediatr Allergy Immunol.* 2010;21:336-44.

56. Apter AJ, Affleck G, Reisine ST, Tennen HA, Barrows E, Wells M, et al. Perception of airway obstruction in asthma: sequential daily analyses of symptoms, peak expiratory flow rate, and mood. *J Allergy Clin Immunol.* 1997;99:605-12.

57. Konradsen JR, Nordlund B, Lidegran M, Pedroletti C, Gronlund H, van Hage M, et al. Problematic severe asthma: a proposed approach to identifying children who are severely resistant to therapy. *Pediatr Allergy Immunol.* 2011;22:9-18.

58. Bush A, Saglani S. Management of severe asthma in children. *Lancet.* 2010;376:814-25.

59. Lang AM, Konradsen J, Carlsen KH, Sachs-Olsen C, Mowinckel P, Hedlin G, et al. Identifying problematic severe asthma in the individual child—does lung function matter? *Acta Paediatr.* 2010;99:404-10.

60. Payne DN, Rogers AV, Adelroth E, Bandi V, Guntupalli KK, Bush A, et al. Early thickening of the reticular basement membrane in children with difficult asthma. *Am J Respir Crit Care Med.* 2003;167:78-82.

61. Fedorov IA, Wilson SJ, Davies DE, Holgate ST. Epithelial stress and structural remodelling in childhood asthma. *Thorax.* 2005;60:389-94.

62. Jenkins HA, Cool C, Szefler SJ, Covar R, Brugman S, Gelfand EW, et al. Histopathology of severe childhood asthma: a case series. *Chest.* 2003;124:32-41.

63. Regamey N, Ochs M, Hilliard TN, Mühlfeld C, Cornish N, Fleming L, et al. Increased airway smooth muscle mass in children with asthma, cystic fibrosis, and non-cystic fibrosis bronchiectasis. *Am J Respir Crit Care Med.* 2008;177:837-43.

64. Barbato A, Turato G, Baraldo S, Bazzan E, Calabrese F, Panizzolo C, et al. Epithelial damage and angiogenesis in the airways of children with asthma. *Am J Respir Crit Care Med.* 2006;174:975-81.

65. Tillie-Leblond I, de Blic J, Jaubert F, Wallaert B, Scheinmann P, Gosset P. Airway remodeling is correlated with obstruction in children with severe asthma. *Allergy.* 2008;63:533-41.

66. Stevenson EC, Turner G, Heaney LG, Schock BC, Taylor R, Gallagher T, et al. Bronchoalveolar lavage findings suggest two different forms of childhood asthma. *Clin Exp Allergy.* 1997;27:1027-35.

67. Johnston SL, Martin RJ. Chlamydophila pneumoniae and Mycoplasma pneumoniae: a role in asthma pathogenesis? *Am J Respir Crit Care Med.* 2005;172:1078-89.

68. O'Byrne PM, Bisgaard H, Godard PP, Pistolesi M, Palmqvist M, Zhu Y, et al. Budesonide/formoterol combination therapy as both maintenance and reliever medication in asthma. *Am J Respir Crit Care Med.* 2005;171:129-36.

69. Lex C, Jenkins G, Wilson NM, Zacharasiewicz A, Erin E, Hansel TT, et al. Does sputum eosinophilia predict the response to systemic corticosteroids in children with difficult asthma? *Pediatr Pulmonol.* 2007;42:298-303.

70. Zhang L, Axelsson I, Chung M, Lau J. Dose response of inhaled corticosteroids in children with persistent asthma: a systematic review. *Pediatrics.* 2011;127:129-38.

71. Cohen J, Postma DS, Douma WR, Vonk JM, De Boer AH, ten Hacken NH. Particle size matters: diagnostics and treatment of small airways involvement in asthma. *Eur Respir J.* 2011;37:532-40.

72. Heller MK, Laks J, Kovesi TA, Ahmet A. Reversal of adrenal suppression with ciclesonide. *J Asthma.* 2010;47:337-9.

73. Simpson JL, Powell H, Boyle MJ, Scott RJ, Gibson PG. Clarithromycin targets neutrophilic airway inflammation in refractory asthma. *Am J Respir Crit Care Med.* 2008;177:148-55.

74. Rodrigo GJ, Neffen H, Castro-Rodriguez JA. Efficacy and safety of subcutaneous omalizumab vs placebo as add-on therapy to corticosteroids for children and adults with asthma: a systematic review. *Chest.* 2011;139:28-35.

75. Busse WW, Morgan WJ, Gergen PJ, Mitchell HE, Gern JE, Liu AH, et al. Randomized trial of omalizumab (anti-IgE) for asthma in inner-city children. *N Engl J Med.* 2011; 364:1005-15.

76. Payne DN, Balfour-Lynn IM, Biggart EA, Bush A, Rosenthal M. Subcutaneous terbutaline in children with chronic severe asthma. *Pediatr Pulmonol.* 2002;33:356-61.

77. Tsai TC, Lu JH, Chen SJ, Tang RB. Clinical efficacy of house dust mite-specific immunotherapy in asthmatic children. *Pediatr Neonatal.* 2010;51:14-8.

78. Pham-Thi N, Scheinmann P, Fadel R, Combebias A, Andre C. Assessment of sublingual immunotherapy efficacy in children with house dust mite-induced allergic asthma optimally controlled by pharmacologic treatment and mite-avoidance measures. *Pediatr Allergy Immunol.* 2007;18:47-57.

79. Coren ME, Rosenthal M, Bush A. The use of cyclosporin in corticosteroid dependent asthma. *Arch Dis Child.* 1997;77:522-3.

80. Rivera-Spoljaric K, Chinchilli VM, Camera LJ, Zeiger RS, Paul IM, Phillips BR, et al. Signs and symptoms that precede wheezing in children with a pattern of moderate-to-severe intermittent wheezing. *J Pediatr.* 2009;154:877-81.e4.

81. Vuillermin P, South M, Robertson C. Parent-initiated oral corticosteroid therapy for intermittent wheezing illnesses in children. *Cochrane Database Syst Rev.* 2006;3: CD005311.

82. Vuillermin PJ, Robertson CF, Carlin JB, Brennan SL, Biscan MI, South M. Parent initiated prednisolone for acute asthma in children of school age: randomised controlled crossover trial. *BMJ.* 2010;340:c843.

83. Bacharier LB, Phillips BR, Zeiger RS, Szefler SJ, Martinez FD, Lemanske RF Jr, et al. Episodic use of an inhaled corticosteroid or leukotriene receptor antagonist in preschool children with moderate-to-severe intermittent wheezing. *J Allergy Clin Immunol.* 2008;122:1127-35.e8.

Difficult Asthma—The Patient's Perspective

Jennifer M Versnel, Liam G Heaney

INTRODUCTION

"For me, it's the constant ache in the back, literally trying to get air into yourself. You are using muscles permanently in your back, and then it's like someone shoving you under the water or putting a cushion over your head. That is scary."[1]

"People don't see me or understand me when I've cried and wept and punched my fist through the wall gasping for another breath, thinking I'm not going to make it this time. I feel like I'm going to die."[2]

Our knowledge about the underlying immunological mechanisms and optimal treatment strategies in asthma has increased substantially in the past three decades. However, for patients with severe disease, which is relatively resistant to currently available therapies, there remains a significant unmet clinical need. Apart from trying to understand the mechanisms which drive severe disease and discover new therapies for these patients, we must also recognize that difficult asthma impacts significantly on people's lives, their family, friends, and those who support their care. Those living with difficult asthma report feelings of fear, anxiety, frustration, embarrassment, marginalization, and discrimination.[1-4]

While national and international guidelines advocate optimal treatment regimens, the evidence base in patients with difficult disease is relatively weak, and these regimens do not always align with what patients consider as important.[5] Understanding the needs and perspectives of patients with difficult asthma will enable the development of more effective education and self-management strategies, which will provide patients with increased understanding of their asthma and make them feel more involved in their treatment. This has the potential to increase adherence, improve symptom control and ultimately health outcomes in this group, with the added potential to reduce significant health costs associated with difficult asthma.

IMPORTANCE OF SPECIALIST CARE

Asthma is traditionally managed in a primary care setting by the general practitioner and this is appropriate for those with mild-to-moderate asthma, where excellent treatment options are currently available. However, as described in Chapter 3, it is important that patients with difficult-to-control asthma are referred to respiratory specialists for a detailed systematic assessment, including access to multidisciplinary services, such as physiotherapy or clinical psychology, where appropriate. This approach ensures that the diagnosis is correct, all symptoms are due to asthma, and identifies comorbidities, which may be impacting on symptom control. Patients may need to be referred to more than one specialist to treat different but inter-related conditions; clinical services which provide a holistic approach to care can help to ensure joined up thinking in terms of overall management (authors' personal communication). Having to take considerable time off work or school can affect a person's ability to hold a job or impact on a child's learning/ability to maintain social relationships (authors' personal communication);[1] specialist centres with multidisciplinary teams can assist by arranging multiple appointments on the same day. Many people report referral to a specialist centre as a turning point for them in gaining greater control over symptoms and exacerbations, however, it can take years and many hospitalizations before they receive the multidisciplinary support they require: "If I wasn't getting specialist care for my asthma, I suspect that one of my four intensive care admissions would have been my last".[1]

Specialist centers often provide patients with a dedicated contact person that they can call if they have concerns or if their asthma worsens. Getting timely advice to adjust a person's medication or the ability to attend the clinic when symptoms worsen could help prevent frequent hospitalizations (authors' personal communication). However, unpredictability of difficult asthma means that even when under the care of respiratory specialists, an exacerbation can result in admission through accident and emergency (A&E) departments. This can, in part, be overcome if people with difficult asthma carry a personalized care plan that has been written by their specialist to ensure optimised treatment in emergency situations (authors' personal communication). People however, report not being taken seriously in emergency departments, these plans being ignored and being given medication that can worsen their situations.[1] This can be extremely stressful for patients and parents (authors' personal communication), "My experience is that once she goes past A&E to the hospital, everything is different. It's just that stumbling block, its like going through a brick wall, once you go through it everything is fine on the other side. The main concern for me is what happens at A&E".[1] There are however examples of excellence we can learn from.

"At the Royal Alexandra, we use a care pathway for children presenting at A&E with acute exacerbation of asthma/wheeze. We also use emergency passports that allow children to have easy access to pediatric expertise and specific management plans related to their condition. Certain children respond better to certain treatments for their asthma, and the emergency passport indicates these to clinicians who are unfamiliar with the child's condition. In addition, clinicians can respond appropriately and in a timely manner to prevent further deterioration of the child. Some children with severe asthma need treatment to be activated quickly and patients and parents are reassured that they have the facility to access care quickly, avoiding long anxious waits in emergency departments."[1]

MANAGEMENT OF DIFFICULT ASTHMA

Research has shown that self-management is often suboptimal in asthma patients and poorly controlled asthma is a significant burden to healthcare system.[5,6] Horne et al. identified the common causes of poor control to be a combination of clinical and behavioral factors.[6] International and national evidence-based guidelines for healthcare professionals advocate optimal control with little impact on lifestyle and minimal side effects; however, in reality, this is difficult to achieve for those affected by severe refractory asthma. This fact increases the importance of identifying any differences which may exist in the perspectives of healthcare professionals and patients, and designing self-management strategies, which are more likely to be adhered to. While clinical factors, such as comorbidities and resistance to therapy play a significant role in the degree of control, behavioral factors such as ability to self-manage, adherence to treatment, and smoking are also important. Aligning clinical management strategies with what patients are seeking in treatment regimens maximizes the potential for improving control of symptoms.[5] Personalized management plans which outline changes to medication when symptoms deteriorate have been shown to be effective in preventing exacerbations, yet observational data has shown that few patients have been provided with such information.[7,8]

Haughney et al. examined the aspects of long-term management that were important to patients with moderate-to-severe asthma (n = 148) by performing a discrete choice experiment where patients rated their preferences by choosing between pairs of hypothetical scenarios.[5] Drawing on previous research, six attributes, which were known to be important to patients were listed together with pairs of choices commonly applied in treatment. These attributes were: "symptom relief provided by your treatment, inhaled steroid dose, use of a written personalized asthma action plan, asthma crisis management, number of different inhalers, and controlling your asthma symptoms".[5] Healthcare professionals manage asthma using national and international guidelines, which rate optimal management in terms of the degree to which symptoms are controlled.[6] However, in this discrete choice experiment, adults with moderate to severe asthma made clear choices with regard to their treatment preferences – the hierarchical choices were (i) a simple treatment regimen with no more than two inhalers, (ii) low doses of inhaled steroids, (iii) having a personalized asthma action plan, (iv) avoiding hospital admission during exacerbations, (v) controlling asthma symptoms, and (vi) relief of symptoms.[5] These results suggest that the patients involved in this study would be prepared to forego increased control of symptoms if this meant the use of fewer inhalers and lower doses of inhaled corticosteroids.[5] This poses a dilemma for healthcare professionals, particularly in the context of the management of difficult asthma which generally requires complex treatment regimens. If patient preferences are for simpler treatment regimens, this may lead to non-adherence and poor outcomes. This means that discussing patient preferences and concerns about treatment regimens is essential and may help to design more effective strategies and improve health outcomes. Regular reviews are important to re-evaluate treatment and discuss patient preferences in order to set realistic goals for asthma management.[6]

Holgate et al. undertook a review of twenty-four European and North American surveys conducted between 1997 and 2003.[9] Whilst these surveys were not specifically designed for difficult asthma, they identified that patients often tolerate high levels of symptoms and had low expectations of their treatment. Despite such symptoms, many underestimated the severity of their condition and believed their asthma to be well controlled. This correlates well with our own data involving eighty-eight patients or carers in eight European countries.[13] The majority of respondents had both asthma and allergy and had lived with their condition(s) for more than five years. Despite nearly half of respondents having symptoms which were not controlled and experiencing high levels of interference with daily life, the majority reported being satisfied or very satisfied with their treatment.[13] If levels of control are to be improved, patient education which addresses poor expectation is essential but is likely to be achieved only when we consider patient perspectives of their condition and treatments.

Another factor, which can impact heavily on management and adherence, is the cost to the patient in countries where patients pay for their medication. Even where treatment is heavily subsidised, patients report having to make choices as to which medicines they take.[10] This can have serious implications for those living with life-threatening conditions and adjusting prescriptions, e.g., to use combination inhalers if appropriate, can reduce the overall cost to the patient. However, unless the issue of cost is identified initially as a potential reason for lack of medication adherence, this issue may not be determined during reviews.

COMPLEX TREATMENT REGIMENS AND SIDE EFFECTS

"I am currently taking 18 different drugs to try and keep some control of my asthma. Of course with all these drugs comes side effects—weight gain, steroid-induced diabetes, potential osteoporosis, to name a few."[1]

"I have been on 40 tablets a day and that is hard. Imagine being sick every day and still having to take 40 pills. That's without all the nebulizers—I have them every four hours."[1]

Comorbidities are common in difficult asthma. Patients often need to take large number of medicines throughout the day to control symptoms, and many are associated with significant side effects.

Concerns around prescribed treatment relate to negative beliefs such as side effects and dependence on large numbers of medicines taken over long periods of time.[6] It is a continual trade off, balancing improved control of symptoms versus the negative impact of side effects, which is a constant struggle for many people and a challenge for healthcare professionals.

"I hate having to take so many pills, potions every day at specific times, it annoys me, it makes me angry. I live by the clock, so I am basically constantly thinking about needing to take my medication, I am always conscious of it."[1]

Despite having concerns, patients may not discuss these with the healthcare professional if they believe that they are faced with no alternative given the severity of the condition. Side effects can present as very visible changes, which affect body image and cause distress. Even if there is little that can be done to reduce these effects, it is important to patients that these are acknowledged and discussed so that they are reassured that other alternatives are not feasible. Whilst patient concerns are often warranted, research has also demonstrated they can be overestimated and based on misunderstandings.[2]

IMPACT OF DIFFICULT ASTHMA ON QUALITY OF LIFE

"My quality of life is non-existent. I know it sounds extreme to a lot of people but I would be prepared to lose an arm or a leg if it meant my asthma would go away."[2]

Living with difficult asthma has enormous physical, emotional, and social impacts on all aspects of a person's life.[9] The majority of people believe asthma is an 'inconvenience' and are unaware that asthma can be a serious and difficult clinical condition—there are frequent reports of men and women, especially in sport, who lead exciting and fulfilling lives despite having asthma and seldom are most people exposed to the reality of living with asthma that is so difficult to manage and people cannot lead normal lives.

"I face daily restrictions in every aspect of my life. I can't visit friends because of their pets, I have problems with barbecues because the smoke sets off my asthma. I find it really difficult to do day-to-day activities on my own—I don't have enough breath to push a trolley around the supermarket. I'm not allowed on an aeroplane and it's

*impossible for me to get travel insurance. Winter is also a problem for me—I can't go
outside because the cold air can set off my asthma" (part of a quote).*[2]

In a survey by Asthma UK in 2009, 98% of children with more difficult asthma
who attended a "Kick Asthma" holiday, reported missing out on something because
of their asthma.[3] In an online survey of children between the ages of 5 and 18, they
reveal feelings of isolation, not being able to participate in sport, being excluded
from school trips, bullying, and missing out on fun. They also battle to keep up with
lessons given the amount of time they are absent.[3]

*"I hate my asthma, it's the worst thing in the world. I can't play as much sport as my
friends and I hate going to hospital."*[3]

*"I was often worried about having an asthma attack in the middle of the night and not
being able to call out for help. I would keep a shoe by my bed and would bang on the
floor for my mother to hear in case I suffered an attack."*[4]

EFFECTS ON FAMILY AND SOCIAL RELATIONSHIPS

The impact of difficult asthma on families is considerable and relationships with
family members strained due to the amount of time those with the condition are
unwell and unable to participate in normal activities. Tasks that the majority of
people take for granted, for example getting dressed, walking, or shopping can be
challenging, and cause frustration and depression. Feelings of vulnerability, fear,
and anxiety are common due to the unpredictability and variable nature of the
condition. Many people with difficult asthma report that they do not leave their home
unaccompanied as they are apprehensive that an exacerbation might leave them
unable to communicate their needs in an emergency situation. An exacerbation can
result in a person being taken to the nearest hospital, which may not be aware of their
personalized treatment and some report frustration with healthcare professionals
not listening to them in such situations (authors' personal communication).

Parents who have a child with difficult asthma can struggle to support the needs
of all their children and maintain a balanced family lifestyle. "When I was a child,
I spent a lot of time in the hospital. My parents were always with me, my sister
resented me, and consequently she lost a lot of time with my parents as well because
they were always by my bedside. In a way, me and my sister have never really had a
relationship. She thinks I took all the time up with me."[1] Additionally parents often
become carers and have to give up work and careers because of the time they need
to devote to support their child through extensive periods away from school and
frequent hospital visits and admissions.

Adults report breakdowns in relationships with partners and friends due to
restrictions on daily life. "The severity of my asthma means that I don't have much

of a social life so I feel very isolated. It's also embarrassing to have to [use] your nebulizer in public. I've lost a lot of friends because of my illness. My relationship with my partner broke down because of my asthma."[2] The majority of people don't give a second thought to the environment before leaving their homes. For some people with difficult asthma, the uncertainly of what triggers they might be exposed to leaves them feeling vulnerable and significantly reduces their ability to socialize. High pollen levels, smoke, pollution, and perfume are just some examples of the many substances, which may cause sudden and difficult exacerbations and can result in hospitalization. "Proceedings had to be halted when I had an asthma attack because of someone's perfume."[2] The implementation of a ban on smoking in public places in many countries has made a significant difference to those with difficult asthma, allowing them to go out to pubs and restaurants and in some cases keep their jobs.[2] However, more needs to be done to support those people in countries where such measures have not been implemented, placing unnecessary restrictions on others.

"In a good month, Jordan will be at school for two out of four weeks. He's now registered with the school at the hospital, which means that any time he's admitted, he'll get two hours of lessons a day. But he has missed so much that he has had to repeat his first year. His primary school was of no help at all, but he has changed schools now and his new teacher has asthma, so things are a lot easier."[2]

The variability of difficult asthma makes planning a holiday stressful; for many people the prohibitive cost of travel insurance, makes travel unaffordable (authors' personal communication). Planning needs to take place months in advance and includes things, such as getting travel insurance, obtaining a 'fitness to fly' certificate, obtaining permission to use a nebulizer on board, researching hospitals abroad, contacting hotels to find out whether they are able to support one's dietary needs and arranging for assistance at airports if the distances one needs to walk are large.[11]

EFFECTS ON EDUCATION AND ABILITY TO WORK

Attending school is an important period in a child's life where they learn to interact socially and develop skills that enable them to fulfill their potential. A research by Staley et al., examined case records of 35 children with difficult allergic asthma and demonstrated that 50% of children had symptoms despite high levels of medication, 40% had poor school attendance, and that there are significant impacts on the economic and emotional functioning of the family unit.[12] Sadly parents and young people report bullying, exclusion from social activities, and difficulties in keeping up with school work due to long absences from school.[1] The side effects of steroids, such as Cushing's Syndrome can affect self-esteem and cause depression – "My son gets teased quite a lot at school. Kids will say, "I don't want to sit next to you, I don't want to catch it." They call him moon face, he gets a pretty hard time of it at school."[1] In a report compiled by Asthma UK, entitled "Missing out", children report that they are either excluded from sports, as teachers are unaware of what they are able to do, or pushed beyond their capabilities without appreciation of the severity of their condition.[3] Parents are often concerned what might happen at school if their child has an asthma attack and many report that their children are not allowed to carry their inhaler with them at all times, which causes unnecessary stress for children and parents. Research conducted by Asthma UK and the National Foundation for Educational Research in 2009 found that around three quarters of teachers in England were unsure of what to do when a child in their class had an asthma attack.[1]

Some adults are so severely affected that even with optimal therapy, they are unable to work or hold down a regular job due to long absences from work or triggers within the workplace. In countries where financial assistance, for example, disability benefits, is available, people report difficulties in accessing such help due to the unpredictability of the condition and the fact that on days they may appear to be well and assessors fail to appreciate how difficult asthma can be. "My life has completely changed in the last year, I was a very busy special-needs classroom assistant, jumping about, I collected the children after school and also had another job. Now I am lucky if I can get washed and dressed in the morning, my life has completely changed for the worse. I loved my job and I'm in the process of maybe having to stop due to ill health."[1]

Many report losing their jobs because of their asthma and this is despite many countries having legislation to protect people with disabilities, however, frequently this is not implemented, leaving people feeling depressed and isolated. "Financially it has been depressing for me. I can't emphasise that more. I worked from 16 and used to start a job and in the three months' probation I would usually have an asthma attack which would put me out of work for a week-ten days and then the employer would let me go... I am just going to have too class myself as ill, but admitting that to yourself at 21 years of age is really difficult. Now I haven't worked for two and a half years."[1]

In general, there is too little awareness that difficult asthma can be a severely disabling condition. "I just feel that people look at you and say, "But there is nothing wrong with you, you have only got asthma," but they don't understand..."[1] Healthcare professionals can help by raising awareness of how disabling asthma can be and provide support to access financial assistance, where appropriate.

CONCLUSION

This chapter attempts to provide a brief insight into the significant obstacles that adults and children with difficult asthma face in their everyday life, and the impact this has on their families and friends. Difficult asthma leaves people feeling anxious, depressed, and fearful, yet the serious effects of difficult asthma are often not appreciated. Many people think of asthma as a relatively mild condition that is easily treated and one which causes minimal interference in daily life. Healthcare professionals, support groups, and policy makers need to continue to raise awareness of this disabling condition and identify ways to support those affected.

Comorbidities are common and add to the complexity of managing difficult asthma. Treatment regimens that demand frequent dosing with multiple therapies, are a constant reminder of a patient's illness as are the many side effects, which often affect body image and feelings of self-worth. Asthma guidelines for healthcare professionals are based on optimizing control of symptoms, which can be extremely challenging. A collaborative concordant approach, taking into consideration the perspectives of patients and identifying any concerns they have is likely to achieve more positive health outcomes for individuals and help to reduce the significant healthcare costs associated with uncontrolled asthma.

For children with difficult asthma, the opportunities many children have to reach their potential may be compromised due to the many absences from school, often for long periods of time. Parents often struggle to balance family life and may be forced to give up their careers in order to care for their child. For those adults who are able to work, they often face discrimination in the workplace and report losing their jobs because of frequent exacerbations despite many countries having policies in place that should protect them.

There is a significant unmet clinical need for patients with difficult asthma, and as well as identifying new treatments, we need to define the best clinical management strategy for assessment and management of this complex patient group. More collaborative approaches, taking into account the perspectives of patients, are likely to reduce the impact of this condition on people's lives and healthcare costs. Whilst this can be time consuming for healthcare professionals in the short-term, the benefits of improved control will outweigh any costs in the longer term.

REFERENCES

1. Fighting for Breath. The hidden lives of people with severe asthma. London: Asthma UK, 2010. Available from URL: www.asthma.org.uk/document.rm?id=1054.
2. Living on a Knife Edge. A powerful and moving account of living with serious symptoms of asthma. London: Asthma UK, 2004. Available from URL: www.asthma.org.uk/document.rm?id=98.
3. Missing Out. Asthma attacks in more ways than one. London: Asthma UK, 2009. Available from URL: www.asthma.org.uk/document.rm?id=751.

4. Severe Asthma in Ireland and Europe - A Patient's Perspective. Asthma Society of Ireland: Asthma Society of Ireland, 2007. Available from URL: http://194.149.76.76/asthma2010/images/uploads/file/publications/Severe-Asthma-Report.pdf.

5. Haughney J, Fletcher M, Wolfe S, Ratcliffe J, Brice R, Partridge MR. Features of asthma management: quantifying the patient perspective. *BMC Pulm Med.* 2007;7:16.

6. Horne R, Price D, Cleland J, Costa R, Covey D, Gruffydd-Jones K, et al. Can asthma control be improved by understanding the patient's perspective? *BMC Pulm Med.* 2007;7:8.

7. Gibson PG, Powell H. Written action plans for asthma: an evidence-based review of the key components. *Thorax.* 2004;59:94-9.

8. Asthma UK. Facts and Stats. [Online] [Cited: 24 February 2011.]

9. Holgate ST, Price D, Valovirta E. Asthma out of control? A structured review of recent patient surveys. *BMC Pulm Med.* 2006;6:S2.

10. Prescription Charges in England. Asthma UK, April 2009. Available from URL: www.asthma.org.uk/document.rm?id=775.

11. Travelling with severe asthma. Asthma UK, December 2009. Available from URL: www.asthma.org.uk/document.rm?id=941.

12. Staley KG, Herzallah R, Pandya H, Humphreys E, Gaillard E. P78 Impact of severe allergic asthma in children: highlighting a role for understanding the family perspective. *Thorax.* 2010;65: A110.

13. Valuing the Patient Perspective. Versnel JM. MPhil Dissertation, University of Cambridge, June 2010.

Comorbidity in Refractory Asthma

Robert Niven

INTRODUCTION

Comorbidity in refractory asthma is often multiple and complex. Other chapters in this book have discussed psychological factors, and as a result this chapter will not address in detail, the comorbidities of anxiety and depression, which are not only common, but almost ubiquitous in a population of chronic disease, threatened by severe and life-threatening exacerbations. Indeed, with the fear of attacks being such a feature, an absence of anxiety and depression might actually be considered abnormal in itself.

Compliance/adherence has also been discussed and the factors related to and responsible for this "comorbidity" will also not be discussed in this chapter further.

To consider comorbidities in detail, the chapter has been separated into sections, and each section reviews the comorbidity and attempts to unravel whether the clinical feature is directly related to the experienced breathlessness symptoms, such as reflux and dysfunctional breathing or is more likely to be considered a complication of therapy, such as diabetes or osteoporosis. Such a classification is complicated by the fact that there is an inevitable interaction between the comorbidity, the asthma, and its therapy, with obesity and reflux esophagitis being clear examples of this.

REFLUX ESOPHAGITIS

Symptoms of reflux are common in individuals with asthma, probably at all levels of severity and there is a clear increased risk of reflux symptoms in this population.[1] The role of reflux in the etiology of asthma symptoms and severity has been long discussed. Mechanisms of impact include neural reflexes between esophageal acid receptors and airway inflammatory responses, in addition to the theoretical impact of possible aspiration of acidic fluid or nonacidic volume reflux into the airway.[2] There remains uncertainty over the relative importance of each of these arguments. Prevalence can only be estimated in severe asthma studies. In a study of primary care data, the general population had a diagnosis of gastroesophageal reflux disease (GERD) recorded for 9.8% of the population, whereas the prevalence was 16.6% in asthma patients.[3] Reviewing the UK severe asthma registry publication, over 30% of patients were prescribed proton pump inhibitors (PPI), with 41% reporting reflux symptoms.[4] In a systematic review from South America, the prevelance of reflux symptoms was reported in 70% of severe asthma patients.[5] In US systematic reviews, the prevalence varied from 12–85% having abnormal esophageal pH monitoring to 50–80% experiencing symptoms.[6,7] These data should not be directly compared, as the diagnostic rigour is different, but the message is clear. It is likely that GERD becomes more frequent with increasing severity of asthma.

Cough as an individual symptom in individuals with airways obstruction can lead to aggressive asthma medical therapy, which may not be warranted on the basis of eosinophilic airway inflammation. Oral corticosteroid therapy at this time might lead to worsening of reflux and the development of a vicious cycle of more therapy; non-response, and further weight gain/worsening reflux.

If there was a causative impact of reflux in asthma severity, then the ultimate test would be the impact of preventing it and the long-term impact on asthma end-points.

However, trials where augmented antireflux therapy has been applied, either medical or surgical, in severe asthma patients have largely shown improvements in reflux symptoms, but unconvincing evidence of improvements in lung function, asthma exacerbations, or other markers of asthma outcome. A Cochrane review failed to find convincing benefit of medical or surgical treatment of reflux on asthma outcome, though the authors reported there may be subgroups of patients who would benefit.[8]

It is likely that asthma therapy encourages the development of reflux and the strong relationship between the two is affected in this direction. Frequent bronchodilator use will probably relax the smooth muscles of the lower esophageal sphincter. Oral steroids and their impact on central obesity increase the abdominal pressure and encourage reflux.

In summary, reflux should be considered as a common comorbidity, treated on its own merit, but at this time, physicians should not consider its treatment as an anti-asthma approach.

DYSFUNCTIONAL BREATHING

Dysfunctional breathing is a name given to a constellation of abnormal patterns of use of respiratory muscles. While not limited to patients with asthma, their presence is best and most frequently described as occurring as a complication of, or in association with evidence of preceding or coexistent asthma. The prevalence and definitions are not easy to quantify, but it is clear that their presence leads to symptoms of disproportionate breathlessness and other somatic symptoms, some of which may be related to physiological changes, such as hypocapnia.[9]

If the pattern of dysfunctional breathing is seen alone in patients with no evidence of underlying genuine respiratory pathology, then we may refer to dysfunctional breathing as being "primary" as in primary hyperventilation. While commonly believed to be the most common form of hyperventilation, Saisch et al., demonstrated that the vast majority of individuals diagnosed with hyperventilation objectively in accident and emergency (A&E) departments, were shown to have known underlying asthma or previously undiagnosed asthma.[10] In an earlier study, DeMeter et al. demonstrated that asthma could be demonstrated in 95% of patients presenting with proven hyperventilation.[11]

HYPERVENTILATION

The most common form of dysfunctional breathing is hyperventilation, which is defined as ventilation above the physiological need. This is usually produced by an increase in respiratory rate, with a near normal tidal volume, resulting in an increased minute volume over and above the physiological need. Different patterns of hyperventilation exist resulting in different clinical syndromes.

Acute (Exercise-induced) Hyperventilation

Prys-Picard et al. demonstrated that a subgroup of patients hyperventilated in response to the "thought of" exercise, with significant immediate increase in respiratory rate and hypocapnea when exercise was commenced (the first minute of a shuttle walk test), but then resolved with increased physiological demand. This pattern was specifically labelled as "anticipatory tachypnea."[12]

Hyperventilation can also be demonstrated towards the latter stages of full cardiopulmonary exercise tests, limiting exercise capacity. These patients have limited exercise capacity caused by their hyperventilation and breathlessness may be the main symptom.

Other triggers of symptoms are many and varied from environmental exposures of irritants, exercise, emotional stress, and in many cases unprovoked. When these triggers induce hyperventilation, the resulting physiological hypocapnea and alkalosis induce the somatic symptoms that are often the hallmark of hyper-ventilation, such as parethesia of hands, circumoral parethesia, chest pain, palpitations, dizziness, and blurred vision.[9] At the same time, there is the sensation of breathlessness, and classical is the feeling, that the patient is unable to take a sufficient inspiratory breath. The latter can result in the sensation referred to as air hunger but may be referred to medically as disproportionate breathlessness, as the degree of perceived breathlessness overwhelms the extent of underlying airway abnormality.[9] Central side effects, such as dizziness, even epileptic events, and tetany can be provoked by severe alkalosis and may result in the individual being initially referred for a neurological opinion.

The prevalence of hyperventilation is unknown. In a primary care population study, Thomas et al.[13] estimated that nearly 30% of patients with a diagnosis of asthma had evidence of hyperventilation, though this study used the Nijmagen questionnaire only to diagnose hyperventilation, and this may be a poor marker of hyperventilation in individuals with asthma, let alone severe asthma.[9,13] In a PhD project, Prys-Picard et al., estimated the prevalence of dysfunctional breathing in a random sample of severe asthma patients of approximately 50% (at least one form of dysfunctional breathing), with nearly 40% having either acute or chronic hyperventilation.[12] The study involved the use of portable plethysmography and measurement of end tidal CO_2 at rest and in response to exercise.

Diagnosing Hyperventilation

Diagnosis is not straight forward, either in an individual or in population studies and often relies on the reporting of the constellation of symptoms experienced when alkalosis ensues.

Historically, physicians tried to reproduce symptoms by inducing hyper-ventilation in the clinic setting and determining whether the symptoms experienced reproduced the patients reported experience. Concerns exist over the safety of this procedure, and it is now best avoided.

The Nijmagen questionnaire is a short specific questionnaire, specifically created to identify individuals with a high index of suspicion of hyperventilation. It is reasonably validated in individuals with no underlying lung disease. However, many of the questions relate closely to symptoms experienced in asthma, and it has been argued and demonstrated that asthma sufferers give high Nijmagen scores even in the absence of hyperventilation. In studies of severe asthma patients, the Nijmagen questionnaire global score did not predict those patients who could be demonstrated objectively to physiologically hyperventilate. Interestingly, in this study, the Nijmagen questionnaire did correlate very strongly with the quality of life questionnaire.[14]

Ideally, diagnosis of acute hyperventilation is made by the demonstration of alkalosis on blood gases after one of the triggers, such as exercise, in response to postural change, or a known trigger performed in the clinic setting. Often, however, the diagnosis is made pragmatically, by the opportunistic measurement of alkalosis when the individual presents with symptom or by an experienced physiotherapist/clinician in response to the clinical syndrome.

Chronic Hyperventilation

In chronic hyperventilation, the patient can be in a near permanent alkalotic or hypo-capneic state. The physiological response continues through sleep and exercise.[15] The condition can usually be diagnosed by simple blood gas measurement at rest or using continuous CO_2 monitoring using cutaneous devices.

Overventilation

This term may be used to describe those individuals who hyperventilate by increasing tidal volume without change in respiratory rate. This tidal volume may be consistently high or might take the form of intermittent normal breaths interspersed with an excess of high volume or sigh breaths.[16]

Treatment of Hyperventilation

Treatment is usually by physiotherapy, with teaching of breathing control mechanisms. While there are many forms, this can take specific reported techniques which include the "Papworth" method.[17] Studies in asthma patients using quality of life responses as the end-point have been positive and there can appear substantial quality of life benefit, with only low number of patients needing to be treated to see a clinical benefit.[18] Thomas et al. reported the number needed to treat of only 3.6,[19] to achieve a clinically meaningful apparent benefit to patients with physiotherapy in patients diagnosed with hyperventilation using the Nijmagen questionnaire.

Studies that have looked for more objective or hard outcome benefits, including exercise tolerance, exercise induced end-tidal CO_2, and even breath hold time have been much more negative.[12,14] This absence of objective markers of improvement, while demonstrating an improvement in asthma-related quality of life markers, questions the mechanism of the benefit reported, which may not be by any real response to the depth or frequency of actual hyperventilation episodes. This supposition is supported by the finding of a close correlation between quality of life end-points and the Nijmagen questionnaire, but an absence of correlation between the latter and objective markers of hyperventilation.[14] As such, patients may report improved quality of life because they feel they have "more control" over the problem, while they have not actually stopped hyperventilating. While at present, it is likely that physiotherapy should be recommended, expectations of treatment should be controlled, so as not to predict the return of normality and particularly normal exercise capacity.

Jack et al. have attempted to try alternative therapies in a cohort of predominantly primary hyperventilating patients. Hypnotherapy, exercise retraining, and exposure to high levels of inhaled CO_2 to desensitize the individual have all shown disappointingly negative results.[15]

OTHER FORMS OF DYSFUNCTIONAL BREATHING

Vocal cord dysfunction (VCD) is the most well known of these but may be less common than previously thought. In one study that systematically and objectively studied the prevalence of VCD found that its prevalence was as low as 1.6%,[5] meaning that no more than 2–3 new cases per year even for the busiest of refractory asthma clinics, were seen.

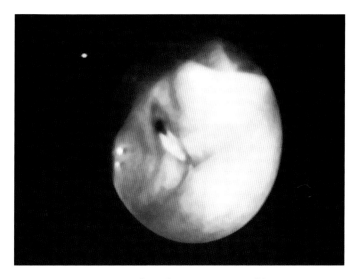

Figure 8-1 Vocal cords in inspiratory adduction.

The term is used to describe the onset of predominantly inspiratory stridor caused by closure of the larynx at vocal cord level due to reflex paradoxical inspiratory adduction of the vocal cords (Figure 8-1).

However, the closure of the larynx can be demonstrated to occur at multiple levels, and it is suggested that the term functional upper airway obstruction may be more accurate.

As with hyperventilation, VCD may occur in either chronic[20] or acute[21] forms, with evidence of continued laryngeal obstruction during sleep witnessed in the chronic form. This indicates that at least in the chronic state, the reflex abnormalities that cause this pattern of disorder are learnt and not under active conscious control. The mechanism is thought to be a hyper-responsiveness of vagally mediated afferent and efferent nerves.[22]

While common in asthma patients, series of clinical cases of VCD have reported the presence of functional upper airway obstruction in individuals who are shown to have no objective evidence of underlying asthma.[23]

Psychological factors do play a part with an excess of psychological abnormalities in people who develop VCD, most clearly demonstrated in previous clinical series being that of separation anxiety. However, many cases exist with no significant psychological abnormality present. Each case must be carefully assessed for the physical, clinical, and psychological factors, and it would be inappropriate to assume that every case has psychological causation.[23]

As an example of physical causation, VCD has been witnessed in athletes, particularly those exposed to airway irritants, such as swimmers (chlorine and chloramines) and speed skaters (cold dry air and possibly ozone).[24] Other localized irritants, such as acid from reflux and other forms of irritants/exercise may be involved in the development of VCD in some cases.

Diagnosis of Vocal Cord Dysfunction

The diagnosis is best made by the clinical visualization of the adducted larynx, or closed upper larynx, while reproducing symptoms. This is usually done by an experienced speech therapist, using a laryngoscope, or possibly a clinician using a bronchoscope. Ear, nose, and throat (ENT) surgeons may miss the condition when investigating stridor, if they are not considering functional changes. Secondly, the clinical pattern of adduction of the vocal cords may need to be induced while visualizing the larynx, and this might mean exposing the individual to the circumstances that induce their symptoms, i.e., exercise, stress, or environmental irritants. In certain specialist centres in Europe, laryngoscopes attached to exercise challenge equipment have been described.[25] More commonly, speech therapists and clinicians act pragmatically to find the most likely mechanism of inducing the attack while in the clinic or bronchoscopy unit.[26]

Other methods of demonstrating the acute development of upper airway obstruction, such as CT scanning,[27] flow volume loops, and even oscillometry have all been attempted, but none appear reliable or preferable to direct visualization.[26]

Treatment of Vocal Cord Dysfunction

Clear benefit of speech therapy has been demonstrated, and this remains the mainstay of therapy. While undergoing speech therapy, addressing underlying triggering factors, including, reflux, psychological factors, and reducing physical triggers (e.g., occupational exposures), if possible, might help, though none has proven efficiency. In those patients who do not respond, other measures have been attempted, including using inspiratory resistance devices,[28] botox injections,[29] and tracheostomy as a last resort.[30] A recent publication[31] has suggested a possible beneficial effect of amitryptilline used in low doses akin to the impact seen in pain therapy. The mechanism of action is presumably through an impact reducing reflex neural arcs.

OTHER PATTERNS OF DYSFUNCTIONAL BREATHING

While most physicians recognize the presence of hyperventilation and VCD in asthma, other patterns of dysfunctional breathing are less well recognized, but failing to consider them may result in over treatment of coexistent asthma.

Prys-Picard et al. described the pattern of breathing at low lung volumes and confirmed that this was caused by displacement of tidal breathing towards end-expiration, rather than any dynamic hyperinflation.[12] The cause is unknown, though these patients may learn to breath at low volume in an attempt to avoid inspiratory cough. The diagnosis can be made using a spirotrac (Figure 8-2) to demonstrate the position of the tidal breath and the degree of expiratory reserve capacity. Attempts have been made to treat it using inspiratory training devices and inhaled analgesic agents.

They also described a temporal disconnect between the thoracic and abdominal components of breathing. This is recognized in emphysema and causes increased work of breathing. However, in severe asthma patients, more extreme asynchrony can be demonstrated and the measurement of asynchrony in a severe asthma population was closely correlated to exercise capacity. This pattern is referred to as thoracoabdominal asynchrony and can be measured using plethysmography (Figure 8-3). No successful treatment has been identified to manage this pattern of dysfunctional breathing.

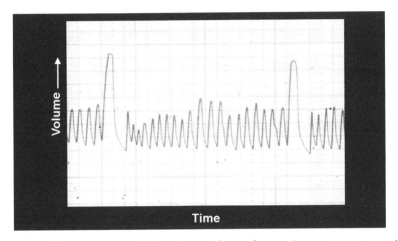

Figure 8-2 Spirotrac showing tidal volume with very low expiratory reserve capacity.

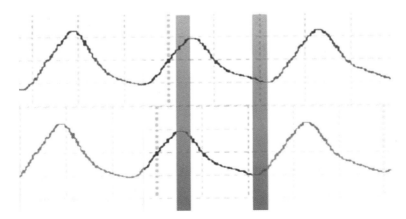

Figure 8-3 Plethysmography of thoracic and abdominal muscles showing asynchrony. The bars are periods of thoraco and abdominal asynchrony.

SUMMARY OF DYSFUNCTIONAL BREATHING

All of these patterns of breathing have been reported alone or in combination in patients with asthma and most notably in severe asthma clinics. Failure to recognize them or to attribute the symptomatic breathlessness they cause to the underlying asthma will potentially result in excess therapy being delivered with associated other comorbidities complicating therapy.

While they may only partially or possibly even fail completely to respond to therapy, diagnosing the condition will allow for more appropriate levels of asthma therapy to be used. Clinicians must consider these comorbidities when assessing patients in severe asthma clinics especially.

OBESITY

The prevalence of obesity in the general population has progressively increased. Recent UK statistics report 24% of men and 30% of women as officially obese, defined by a body mass index (BMI) >30.[32] The prevalence of obesity in asthma patients has probably risen in parallel and a causal effect has been suggested,[33] with data from the recent UK registry, reporting on patients attending severe/refractory asthma clinics to have a mean BMI within the total population being 28, with approximately 40% of individuals fulfilling the criteria of officially obese.[4]

Obesity like reflux and dysfunctional breathing follows the theme of the chapter of being a comorbidity in which the cause and effect component may both be equally powerful and difficult to separate.

Obesity has been reported as causing airway obstruction in the absence of airway inflammation, airway reactivity, and airway inflammation directly as consequence of the obesity.[34] With all of these aspects of asthma being variably reported as a consequence of obesity and the degree of obesity being an inevitable consequence of oral steroid use and reduced inactivity of refractory asthma, the separation of cause and effect is impossible to clarify. In addition, obesity alone like dysfunctional breathing results in nonasthmatic breathlessness and itself may provoke excess therapy.

Todd et al. reported an increase in airway inflammation and a reduced residual capacity in obese individuals and argued that this was the cause of measurable worsened reactivity.[34]

When the majority of excess therapy is oral corticosteroid, the subsequent Cushingoid type central obesity can set up a vicious cycle of worsening obesity-related breathlessness superimposed on asthma. In addition, there are reports of obese asthma patients having an attenuated response to inhaled corticosteroids.[35] As a result, finding mechanisms for objectively tailoring the steroid dose to patients has major beneficial potential in this subgroup of patients.

Obesity also interacts with a number of other comorbidities, for example, it worsens reflux esophagitis and interacts with certain patterns of dysfunctional breathing, resulting in a complex interaction of potential factors.

Other obesity related comorbidities may then also be associated with presence of refractory asthma. For example, Julien et al. have reported that up to 88% of severe asthma patients may have obstructive sleep apnea compared to 31% in a control population.[36]

Losing weight in the presence of oral corticosteroids is challenging even for the most motivated patient. Clinical experience would indicate that if achieved it can result in significant overall benefit, not least in exercise capacity, though trial evidence of this in asthma is limited.

Agents or procedures to effect weight loss may be considered and include medical agents or bariatric surgery. Such approaches often need localized expertise and currently centers specializing in managing asthma may not be found in the same hospitals as those providing obesity services, leaving challenges over shared management.

OSTEOPOROSIS

Many severe asthma patients also suffer or are at risk of osteoporosis. There is controversy over the role of inhaled steroids and the risk of osteoporosis in adults. There are limited studies, which suggest a positive relationship between osteoporosis and even low-dose inhaled steroids,[37] while other studies fail to support this hypothesis.[38,39] The biological plausibility of a direct effect of low-moderate dose inhaled steroids alone as a cause of established osteoporosis seems remote. However, there is little to doubt that those patients requiring frequent courses or regular oral corticosteroids are at increased risk.[40] In the recent UK severe asthma registry study, the mean bone density in all patients attending the three centers where this was measured routinely, T score mean was –0.64 in the spine (L1 to L4) and –0.26 in the femoral neck. These values are relatively reassuring with therefore the majority of patients having normal bone density, despite 40% of patients in this study being on maintenance oral steroids and with a median inhaled steroid dose of 2,000 µg of BDP equivalent for all patients.

Steroids may not be the only cause of osteoporosis in asthma, with reduced physical capacity reducing the osteoblastic activity, similar to the mechanism argued in cystic fibrosis. Recent evidence has suggested that asthma patients may be more prone to vitamin D deficiency.

Current guidance recommends the use of biphosphonates prophylactically in those patients taking moderate doses of oral steroids on a daily basis or frequent bursts of oral steroids. However, new evidence on persistent bone fragility in patients taking biphosphonates and the availability of dexa bone scanning, might support centers to adopt a more observatory and targeted approach and only treat those with established osteoporosis at presentation or those showing evidence of excess loss of bone density on serial scanning. Development of femoral, vertebral, or even rib fractures will have potential severe adverse effect on the quality of life of asthma patients, indeed rib and vertebral fractures may have impact on short- and long-term breathlessness and exercise capacity in patients.

In addition to osteoporosis, a rare complication of oral corticosteroids is avascular necrosis of the hip and may be seen more frequently in severe asthma clinics than may be expected.

DIABETES

Diabetes as a comorbidity is likely to be purely related to the active or historic use of oral corticosteroids. In a population study, the prevalence of diabetes in the general population in Europe was 7.8% and 8.4% in asthma diagnosed individuals.

In a population where a high proportion of patients are on maintenance oral steroids, the prevalence of diabetes is likely to be much higher, although published evidence of the prevalence of diabetes in oral steroid dependent asthma is sparse,[41] and there is none or little evidence to support an impact of high-dose inhaled steroids.[42]

While it is likely that there is a link between treatment for severe asthma and the onset of diabetes, there is established evidence that the presence of diabetes increases the risk of mortality associated with severe asthma patients[43] and the risk of an adverse outcome in terms of future hospitalization or need for A&E attendance.[44]

When it occurs, the management should be as for non-asthma related diabetes, but there may be an increased consideration of the use of steroid-sparing therapies to make it easier to manage diabetes and reduce long-term complications of diabetes. Poorly controlled diabetes in asthma is likely to result in an increased risk and cost of managing secondary complications, including cerebrovascular, cardiovascular, peripheral vascular, renal, and ocular complications. The health-related economic costs of steroid-induced diabetes in severe asthma is completely unknown.

Another outstanding question is whether patients on oral steroids should be subjected to routine screening for diabetes, including annual glucose tolerance tests as in the cystic fibrosis population, which has a similar increased risk. This is not yet routinely practiced, but it could be argued that early diagnosis would aid in long-term management and reduced complications.

EYE DISEASE

Inhaled steroids have been associated with the development of cataracts and while again these are much more likely to occur in patients on frequent or maintenance oral corticosteroids, they are frequent in patients attending severe asthma clinics.

A meta-analysis demonstrated an increase risk of 25% for each 1,000 µg per day increase in the dose of beclomethasone equivalent inhaled steroid dose.[45]

Glaucoma risk is also increased in asthma patients on oral steroids.[46]

Regular eye examinations should be recommended for all severe asthma patients on maintenance oral corticosteroids irrespective of age.

BRONCHIECTASIS

Bronchiectasis is arguably the most underdiagnosed respiratory condition with prevalence rates as high as 35% in severe asthma studies[47] and 50% in chronic obstruction pulmonary disease (COPD) studies, being reported from routine use of high resolution computed tomography (HRCT) scanning. The current rates of reported bronchiectasis, higher than those seen in early systematic reviews (3 and 13%, respectively from London and Belfast cohorts), may represent a change in diagnostic criteria.[48,49]

However, it is clear that there are no uniformly agreed radiological criteria for the diagnosis, and a recent consensus study has suggested that the diagnosis should only be made when there is concordance of appropriate clinical symptoms with typical radiological features of bronchial dilatation, lack of tapering, bronchial thickening, and mucous plugging. These radiological features are very similar to some of those seen in asthma (bronchial dilation, thickening, and plugging), and hence there is likely to be a significant degree of diagnostic overlap (Holme; unpublished data).

Due to this overlap, bronchiectasis might not be considered a comorbidity but more of a different phenotype of severe asthma. However, clinical awareness of this phenotype is critical as it is unlikely that bronchiectasis phenotype will respond to anti-eosinophilic therapy including oral corticosteroids. Again, failure to consider the diagnosis could result in excessive therapy for "refractory" symptoms and subsequent referral to a severe asthma clinic. Consequently, the true prevalence of bronchiectasis in severe asthma may be overestimated and a result of diagnostic failure.

Once the diagnosis is confirmed, therapeutic trials of hypertonic saline[50,51] and low-dose macrolides for their immunemodulatory and possibly mucolytic properties[52] are most likely to be successful. However, the most recent guidance for bronchiectasis still questions the evidence base for the benefit of macrolides.[53]

Hypertonic saline has proven benefit in bronchiectasis, but as there is a risk of coexistent bronchial reactivity and bronchiectasis in the population referred to refractory asthma clinics, a pre-treatment test dosing of hypertonic saline in the clinic is recommended. Most of the evidence of efficacy has been done using 7% saline, nebulized daily initially.[50,51] If the forced expiratory volume in 1 second (FEV_1) falls by less than 10% from baseline during the challenge process (challenge is done using spirometery pre- and post-observerd dosing with hypertonic saline), patients may then be provided with home, 2–3 month trial of daily therapy.

Alternative treatments with mucolytics, such as cysteines are also possible, but evidence of persisting effect is limited.

Treatment should aim to break the cycle of recurrent infection and further airway damage and mucus retention.

When bronchiectasis is documented and possibly routinely within refractory asthma clinics, functional antibody deficiency should be tested. There is a high prevalence of functional antibody deficiency in severe asthma, and recent data suggest this may be related to severity as defined by lower lung function at presentation, within this population (Wardman et al.; unpublished data).

ALLERGIC BRONCHOPULMONARY ASPERGILLOSIS AND SEVERE ASTHMA WITH FUNGAL SENSITIZATION

Allergic bronchopulmonary aspergillosis (ABPA) is a long accepted syndrome associated with central bronchiectasis, high IgE and IgG antibodies to *Aspergillus* or other fungi, and eosinophilia. Specific diagnostic criteria are long established and studies have confirmed the benefit of antifungal therapy in this population.

Recently, Niven and Denning proposed a second syndrome labeled severe asthma with fungal sensitization (SAFS). This relied on a prediagnosis of severe asthma and required the presence of fungal sensitization confirmed by either positive radioallergosorbent tests (RASTs) to specific fungal allergens or skin prick test positivity. ABPA patients were excluded to exclude overlap.[54]

The importance of this syndrome is its high prevalence in certain severe asthma clinics,[45] which may be geographically and environmentally driven but results in a high morbidity and health-related resource utilization. There is also a clear and long-established evidence of the poor prognostic impact of fungal sensitization, with studies documenting an increased risk of hospitalization, high-risk attacks, and mortality in those sensitized to fungal allergens compared to those nonallergic.[54,55] The prevalence of fungal allergy showed marked variation within the UK severe asthma registry study, with prevalence rates below 20% in Leicester and Belfast and over 40 and 50% in London and Manchester, respectively. In a single center study, fungal allergy was also associated with the presence of bronchiectasis but not restricted to the central form required for a label of ABPA.[47]

The same authors produced evidence of significant benefit of treating these patients with antifungal therapy, showing large benefits in terms of quality of life (0.81 improvements over placebo) in an eight-month therapy study.[56]

The hypothesis is that patients with a degree of airway damage or chronic inflammation become colonized with fungal allergens, which are not cleared. In those patients with allergy to these allergens, a chronic localized allergic response ensues, which only poorly responds to anti-inflammatory therapy. Antifungal therapy at least reduces the extent of colonization and clinical benefit ensues by a reduced allergic response, which can be supported by rapid and large falls in total and RAST specific IgE levels.[56]

This hypothesis of fungal colonization has been supported by studies from Leicester, which have demonstrated that those patients with fungal sensitization can be shown to have fungal presence in sputum samples using advanced culture techniques when compared to those patients with similar severe asthma who are not so sensitized. These data have only been submitted as scientific abstracts to date and await formal publication (Wardlaw; unpublished data).

Treatment is complicated by significant and sometimes dangerous interactions between itraconazole and inhaled steroids, with severe Cushingoid and adrenal suppression reactions being reported. Indeed this has led some to question the mechanism of action of the benefit of itraconazole seen in placebo-controlled trials. At the time of writing this chapter, studies assessing the efficacy of alternative anti-fungal agents, which do not interact with inhaled steroids, are awaited.

Certainly at this time, it is recommended that use of antifungal drugs is restricted to specialist centers with experience in their use. Specifically, there is a need to monitor drug levels, taper inhaled steroids when using itraconazole, monitor liver function, and total and specific RAST levels as immunological markers of response. Currently, the prevalence of itraconazole resistant strains and failure to respond to therapy is between 10 and 20%, which highlights a need for more aggressive mycological investigation, possibly, including bronchoscopy to obtain lower respiratory tract samples. A dedicated fungal culture laboratory may be advantageous.

RHINITIS/THE UPPER AIRWAY

The upper and lower airways are connected with both neural interconnections and share chemical/inflammatory receptors. Secondly, the exposure to allergens occurs in both parts of the airway with the only difference being the potential removal of large allergens in the upper airway, preventing lower airways from similar exposure.

The prevalence of allergic rhinitis in asthma and allergy clinics is high. In the ONEAIR study, which examined the prevalence of asthma and rhinitis attending European allergy clinics, the prevalence of rhinitis at presentation was as high as 89%.[57] While this prevalence seems very high in a South American population of severe asthma patients, a similar high prevalence of rhinitis (91%) was reported in a review of patients attending a severe asthma clinic.[5] In the UK BTS registry publication of those with definitive responses, 30% reported seasonal rhinitis, 38% perennial rhinitis, 15% previous nasal surgery, and 14% nasal polyps.[4]

In terms of the importance of the coexistence of asthma and rhinitis, many specialists have recommended a single airway approach suggesting that rhinitis should not even be considered a comorbidity, more an accepted aspect of asthma, which may express itself variably both in severity and in temporal cycles. The latter argument would ensure that the upper airway is always considered as a part of the total refractory asthma package.

There is evidence of a link between the presence of rhinitis and the apparent "severity or refractoriness" of the asthma. It has been previously suggested that the presence of comorbid rhinitis results in a greater likelihood of patients attending emergency care services,[58,59] though other studies have not shown allergic rhinitis to be a predictor of severe asthma,[60] or have suggested there is a gender impact with a more predictive effect for asthma severity in women alone.[61] In the previously mentioned ONEAIR study, presence of rhinitis was actually inversely related to asthma severity.[57] In a study by Cicillo et al.,[62] severity of bronchial hyper-reactivity was predicted by the duration of allergic rhinitis (OR adjusted 5.4) as well as tree and house dust mite sensitization and low baseline FEV_1.

In a study by Agondi et al., treatment of rhinitis was associated with a marked improved in bronchial reactivity after nearly three months of therapy.[63] However, comparing different treatment approaches is more controversial. In terms of relative effectiveness of medical or surgical approaches, trials have tended to support a longer lasting effect of medical over surgical therapy.[64] Medical therapy was associated with more marked improvements in lower airway inflammatory markers and airway physiology when compared to a surgical approach.

The role of omalizumab in treating asthma and coexistent allergic rhinitis has shown moderate success, but, in general, it is likely that similar to the lower airways, the upper airway probably has different phenotypes with variable allergy, inflammatory, and reactive components. A simple single therapy approach is therefore, not likely to work.

CONCLUSION

This chapter alone has touched on the impact of VCD, reflux esophagitis, and rhinitis. Refractory asthma services need to work closely with upper airway clinicians, surgical, medical, and speech and language therapists.

REFERENCES

1. Sontag SJ, O'Connell S, Khandelwal S, Greenlee H, Schnell T, Nemchausky B, et al. Asthmatics with gastroesophageal reflux: long term results of a randomised trial of medical and surgical antireflux therapies. *Am J Gastroenterol.* 2003;98:987-99.
2. McCallister JW, Parsons JP, Mastronarde JG. The relationship between gastroesophageal reflux and asthma: an update. *Ther Adv Respir Dis.* 2011;5:143-50.
3. Cazzola M, Calzetta L, Bettoncelli G, Novelli L, Cricelli C, Rogliani P. Asthma and comorbid medical illness. *Eur Respir J.* 2011;38:42-9.
4. Heaney LG, Brightling CE, Menzies-Gow A, Stevenson M, Niven RM: British Thoracic Society Difficult Asthma Network. Refractory asthma in the UK: cross-sectional findings from a UK multicentre registry. *Thorax.* 2010;65:787-94.
5. Bisaccioni C, Aun MV, Cajuela E, Kalil J, Agondi RC, Giavina-Bianchi P. Comorbidities in severe asthma: frequency of rhinitis, nasal polyposis, gastroesophageal reflux

disease, vocal cord dysfunction and bronchiectasis. *Clinics (Sao Paulo)*. 2009;64: 769-73.

6. Havemann BD, Henderson CA, El-Serag HB. The association between gastroesophageal reflux and asthma: a systematic review. *Gut.* 2007;56:1654-64.

7. Thakkar K, Boatright RO, Gilger MA, El-Serag HB. Gastroesophageal reflux and asthma in children: a systematic review. *Pediatrics.* 2010;125:e925-30.

8. Gibson PG, Henry RL, Coughlan JL. Gastroesophageal reflux treatment for asthma in adults and children. *Cochrane Database Syst Rev.* 2003;CD001496.

9. Morgan MD. Dysfunctional breathing in asthma: is it common, identifiable and correctable? *Thorax.* 2002;57:1131-5.

10. Saisch SG, Wessely S, Gardner WN. Patients with acute hyperventilation presenting to an inner-city emergency department. *Chest.* 1996;110:952-7.

11. Demeter SL, Cordasco EM. Hyperventilation syndrome and asthma. *Am J Med.* 1986; 81:989-94.

12. Prys-Picard CO, Niven R. Dysfunctional breathing in patients with asthma. *Thorax.* 2008;63:568.

13. Thomas M, McKinley RK, Freeman E, Foy C. Prevalence of dysfunctional breathing in patients treated for asthma in primary care: cross-sectional survey. *BMJ.* 2001;322:1098-100.

14. Stanton AE, Vaughn P, Carter R, Bucknall CE. An observational investigation of dysfunctional breathing and breathing control therapy in a problem asthma clinic. *J Asthma.* 2008;45:758-65.

15. Jack S, Rossiter HB, Pearson MG, Ward SA, Warburton CJ, Whipp BJ. Ventilatory responses to inhaled carbon dioxide hypoxia and exercise in idiopathic hyperventilation. *Am J Respir Crit Care Med.* 2004;170:118-25.

16. Prys-Picard CO, Kellett F, Niven RM. Disproportionate breathlessness associated with deep sighing breathing in a patient presenting with difficult to treat asthma. *Chest.* 2006;130:1723-5.

17. Holloway EA, West RJ. Integrated breathing and relaxation training (the Papworth method) for adults with asthma in primary care: a randomised controlled trial. *Thorax.* 2007;62:1039-42.

18. Thomas M, McKinley RK, Mellor S, Watkin G, Holloway E, Scullion J, et al. Breathing exercises for asthma: a randomised controlled trial. *Thorax.* 2009;64:55-61.

19. Thomas M, McKinley RK, Freeman E, Foy C, Prodger P, Price D. Breathing retraining for dysfunctional breathing in asthma: a randomised controlled trial. *Thorax.* 2003;58:110-5.

20. Warburton CJ, McL Niven R, Higgins BG, Pickering CA. Functional upper airways obstruction: two patients with persistent symptoms. *Thorax.* 1996;51:965-6.

21. Niven RM, Roberts T, Pickering CA, Webb AK. Functional upper airways obstruction presenting as asthma. *Respir Med.* 1992;86:513-6.

22. Ayres JG, Gabbott PL. Vocal cord dysfunction and laryngeal hyperresponsiveness: a function of altered autonomic balance? *Thorax.* 2002;57:284-5.

23. Newman KB, Mason UG, Schmaling KB. Clinical features of vocal cord dysfunction. *Am J Respir Crit Care Med.* 1995;152:1382-6.

24. Elers J, Pederesen L, Backer V. Asthma in elite athletes. *Expert Rev Respir Dis.* 2011; 5:343-51.

25. Heimdal JH, Roksund OD, Halvorsen T, Skadberg BT, Olofsson J. Continuous laryngoscopy exercise test: a method for visualizing laryngeal dysfunction during exercise. *Laryngoscope.* 2006;116:52-7.

26. Ayres JG, Mansur AH. Vocal cord dysfunction considering the total airway. *Am J Respir Crit Care Med.* 2011;184:2-3.

27. Low K, Lau KK, Holmes P, Crossett M, Vallance N, Phyland D, et al. Abnormal vocal cord function in difficult-to-treat asthma. *Am J Respir Crit Care Med.* 2011;184:50-6.

28. Archer GJ, Hoyle JL, McCluskey A, Macdonald J. Inspiratory vocal cord dysfunction, a new approach to treatment. *Eur Resp ir J.* 2000;15:617-8.

29. Ekbom DC, Garrett CG, Yung KC, Johnson FL, Billante CR, Zealear DL, et al. Botulinum toxin injections for new onset bilateral vocal fold impairment in adults. *Laryngoscope.* 2010;120:758-63.

30. Goldstein R, Bright J, Jones SM, Niven RM. Severe vocal cord dysfunction resistant to all current therapeutic interventions. *Respir Med.* 2007;101:857-8.

31. Varney V, Parnell H, Evans J, Cooke N, Lloyd J, Bolton J. The successful treatment of vocal cord dysfunction with low-dose amitriptyline-including literature review. *J Asthma Allergy.* 2009;2:105-10.

32. The Health and Social Care Information Centre. Statistics on obesity, physical activity and diet: England, 2010. Available from URL: http://www.ic.nhs.uk/webfiles/publications/opad10/Statistics_on_Obesity_Physical_Activity_and_Diet_England_2010.pdf.

33. Obesity: preventing and managing the global epidemic. Report of a WHO consultation. *World Health Organ Tech Rep Ser.* 2000;894:1-253.

34. Todd DC, Armstrong S, D'Silva L, Allen CJ, Hargreave FE, Parameswaran K. Effect of obesity on airway inflammation: a cross-sectional analysis of body mass index and sputum cell counts. *Clin Exp Allergy.* 2007;37:1049-54.

35. Peters-Golden M, Swerm A, Bird SS, Hustad CM, Grant E, Edelman JM. Influence of body mass index on the response to asthma controller agents. *Eur Respir J.* 2006;27:495-503.

36. Julien JY, Martin JG, Ernst P, Olivenstein R, Hamid Q, Lemière C, et al. Prevalence of obstructive sleep apnea-hypopnea in severe versus moderate asthma. *J Allergy Clin Immunol.* 2009;124:371-6.

37. Bonala SB, Reddy BM, Silverman BA, Bassett CW, Rao YA, Amara S, et al. Bone mineral density in women with asthma on long term inhaled corticosteroid therapy. *Ann Allergy Asthma Immunol.* 2000;85:495-500.

38. Pasaoglu G, Gok H, Mungan D, Sonel B, Yalcin P, Misirligil Z. Does the combination of inhaled steroids with long acting beta2 agonists decrease the risk for osteoporosis? A 1-year prospective follow-up study. *Rheumatol Int.* 2006;27:141-6.

39. El O, Gulbahar S, Ceylan E, Ergor G, Sahin E, Senocak O, et al. Bone mineral density in asthmatic patients using low dose inhaled glucocorticosteroids. *J Investig Allergol Clin Immunol.* 2005;15:57-62.

40. Villareal MS, Klaustermeyer WB, Hahn TJ, Gordon EH. Osteoporosis in steroid-dependent asthma. *Ann Allergy Asthma Immunol.* 1996;76:369-72.

41. Lieberman P, Patterson R, Kunske R. Complications of long-term steroid therapy for asthma. *J Allergy Clin Immunol.* 1972;49:329-36.

42. Faul JL, Wilson SR, Chu JW, Canfield J, Kuschner WG. The effect of an inhaled corticosteroid on glucose control in type 2 diabetes. *Clin Med Res.* 2009;7:14-20.

43. Watson L, Turk F, James P, Holgate ST. Factors associated with mortality after an asthma admission: a national United Kingdom database analysis. *Respir Med.* 2007;101:1659-64.

44. Miller MK, Lee JH, Blanc PD, Pasta DJ, Gujrathi S, Barron H, et al. TENOR risk score predicts health care in adults with severe or difficult-to-treat-asthma. *Eur Respir J.* 2006;28:1145-55.

45. Weatherall M, Clay J, James K, Perrin K, Shirtcliffe P, Beasley R. Dose-response relationship of inhaled corticosteroids and cataracts: a systematic review and meta-analysis. *Respirology.* 2009;14:983-90.

46. Clarke E, Suissa S LeLorier J. Association of inhaled corticosteroids use with cataract extraction in elderly patients. *JAMA.* 1998;280:539-43.

47. Menzies D, Holmes L, McCumesky G, Prys-Picard C, Niven R. Aspergillus sensitisation is associated with airflow limitation and bronchiectasis in severe asthma. *Allergy.* 2011;66:679-85.

48. Heaney LG, Conway E, Kelly C, Johnston BT, English C, Stevenson M, et al. Predictors of therapy resistant asthma: outcome of a systematic evaluation protocol. *Thorax.* 2003;58:561-6.

49. Robinson DS, Campbell DA, Durham SR, Pfeffer J, Barnes PJ, Chung KF; Asthma and Allergy Research Group of the National Heart and Lung Institute. Systematic assessment of difficult-to-treat-asthma. *Eur Respir J.* 2003;22:478-83.

50. Kellett F, Redfern J, Niven RM. Evaluation of nebulised hypertonic saline (7%) as an adjunct to physiotherapy in patients with stable bronchiectasis. *Respir Med.* 2005;99:27-31.

51. Kellett F, Robert NM. Nebulised 7% hypertonic saline improves lung function and quality of life in bronchiectasis. *Respir Med.* 2011;105:1831-5.

52. Kanoh S, Rubin BK. Mechanisms of action and clinical application of macrolides as immunomodulatory medications. *Clin Microbiol Rev.* 2010;23:590-615.

53. Pasteur MC, Bilton D, Hill AT; British Thoracic Society Bronchiectasis non-CF Guideline Group. British Thoracic Society guideline for non-CF bronchiectasis. *Thorax.* 2010;65:i1-58.

54. Denning DW, O'Driscoll BR, Hogaboam CM, Bowyer P, Niven RM. The link between fungi and severe asthma: a summary of the evidence. *Eur Respir J.* 2006;27:615-26.

55. O'Driscoll BR, Hopkinson LC, Denning DW. Mold sensitization is common amongst patients with severe asthma requiring multiple hospital admissions. *BMC Pulm Med.* 2005;5:4-9.

56. Denning DW, O'Driscoll BR, Powell G, Chew F, Atherton GT, Vyas A, et al. Randomised controlled trial of oral antifungal treatment for severe asthma with fungal sensitisation: The Fungal Asthma Sensitisation Trail (FAST) study. *Am J Crit Care Med.* 2009;179:11-8.

57. Navarro A, Valero A, Juliá B, Quirce S. Coexistence of asthma and allergic rhinitis in adult patients attending allergy clinics: ONEAIR study. *J Investig Allergol Clin Immunol.* 2008;18:233-8.

58. Lasmar LM, Camargos PA, Ordones AB, Gaspar GR, Campos EG, Ribeiro GA. Prevalence of allergic rhinitis and its impact on the use of emergency care services in a group of children and adolescents with moderate to severe persistent asthma. *J Pediatr (Rio J).* 2007;83:555-61.

59. Ponte EV, Franco R, Nascimento HF, Souza-Machado A, Cunha S, Barreto ML, et al. Lack of control of severe asthma is associated with co-existence of moderate-to-severe rhinitis. *Allergy.* 2008;63:564-9.

60. de Marco R, Marcon A, Jarvis D, Accordini S, Almar E, Bugiani M, et al. European Community Respiratory Health Survey Therapy Group. Prognostic factors of asthma severity: a 9-year international prospective cohort study. *J Allergy Clin Immunol.* 2006;117:1249-56.

61. Cazzoletti L, Marcon A, Corsico A, Janson C, Jarvis D, Pin I, et al. Asthma severity according to Global Initiative for asthma and its determinants: an international study. *Int Arch Allergy Immunol.* 2010;151:70-9.

62. Cirillo I, Pistorio A, Tosca M, Ciprandi G. Impact of allergic rhinitis on asthma: effects on bronchial hyperreactivity. *Allergy.* 2009;64:439-44.

63. Agondi RC, Machado ML, Kalil J, Giavina-Bianchi P. Intranasal corticosteroid administration reduces nonspecific bronchial hyperresponsiveness and improves asthma symptoms. *J Asthma.* 2008;45:754-7.

64. Ragab S, Scadding GK, Lund VJ, Saleh H. Treatment of chronic rhinosinusitis and its effects on asthma. *Eur Resp J.* 2006;28:68-74.

Molecular and Immunological Basis for Severe Therapy-resistant Asthma

9

Ian M Adcock, Kian F Chung

INTRODUCTION

Degranulated mast cells, an infiltration of eosinophils, and an increased number of activated type 2 T helper (Th2) cells represents an asthma-specific pattern of airway inflammation.[1] It is also becoming clear that subsets of patients with asthma exist,[2,3] and that particular types of inflammatory phenotypes may define the response to particular selective therapies.[2,4]

The most successful anti-inflammatory treatment for asthma is corticosteroids (CS). The advent of topical inhaled corticosteroids (ICS) in the 1970s was a major advance on systemic corticosteroids, which were first introduced in the 1950s resulting in the greater use of these preventers.[5] The routine use of ICS to prevent airway inflammation in combination with relievers, such as β_2-agonists, which help the airway smooth muscle to relax after contraction[6] have led to further improvements in outcomes of asthma. Unfortunately, in a small but significant minority (5–10%) of cases, CS are ineffective.[7-9] These treatment-refractory patients carry a higher burden of costs (economic, morbidity and mortality) compared to nonsevere patients.[8]

Other chapters in this book have defined various aspects of refractory asthma, and this chapter deals with some of the immune and molecular events that occur in these patients and may affect the patient's ability to respond to ICS and oral CS. Indeed, this category of patients have also been labeled as therapy-resistant or refractory asthma.[10,11] Importantly, this relative steroid insensitivity is seen to a greater or lesser extent in most chronic inflammatory diseases as well as in severe asthma.[9] The authors believe that a greater understanding of the mechanisms of CS action and their ineffectiveness in some patients will lead to the development of new drugs particularly in situations where current anti-inflammatory therapies are suboptimal.[12] The aim of this review is to discuss the underlying molecular and immunological basis of severe refractory asthma that could be involved in interfering with the mechanisms of CS action, and how these are thought to be altered in severe refractory asthma. The distinct patterns of inflammation found in refractory asthma may also contribute to the failure to respond, as the drivers of disease subphenotypes may, in themselves, be CS refractory.

MECHANISM OF CORTICOSTEROID ACTION

ICS alone, or particularly in combination with long-acting β_2-agonists (LABAs), are effective in treating symptoms, reducing exacerbations, and improving lung function in most asthmatics.[6,13] These effects of ICS are mediated through alleviating the underlying chronic inflammation present in asthma.

CS, delivered orally or topically, are rapidly absorbed by the body and quickly diffuse across the cell membrane into the cytoplasm where they bind to and activate a specific receptor [glucocorticoid receptor (GR)].[14] GR is present in varying amounts in all resident and infiltrating cells within the airways and lungs, which may account for the effectiveness of ICS in controlling asthmatic inflammation.[15] Activated GR translocates to the nucleus where it has two major roles: it can bind to DNA at specific glucocorticoid response elements (GREs) as a homodimer and activate anti-inflammatory genes (transactivation), or acting as a monomer, GR recruits transcriptional repressor proteins to the promoter regions of inflammatory genes thereby switching off their expression.[14] In the latter case, the most common targets for tethering of monomeric activated GR are the proinflammatory transcription factors activator protein (AP)-1 and nuclear factor κB (NF-κB) which control the expression of many inflammatory and immune genes.[16]

The primary form of GR is GRα, although other forms exist.[17,18] These N- or C-terminally truncated forms may have distinct functions and/or activities and have been postulated to modulate CS activity in treatment-refractory diseases.[17,18] The best example of this is GRβ which has a divergent C-terminal resulting in GRβ being unable to correctly bind to CS or activate gene expression and can act as a dominant negative modulator of GRα.[19] Enhanced expression of GRβ has been reported in some patients with refractory asthma,[19,20] possibly due to expression by proinflammatory cytokines, such as tumor necrosis factor-α (TNF-α) and interleukin-1 (IL-1).[17,21] However, the role of GRβ remains controversial, as its proteins levels compared to that of GRα in these patients may not be enough to allow suppression of GRα actions.[20]

Gene induction, whether driven by NF-κB or by activated GR, requires the action of transcriptional coactivators. These coactivators are modular proteins, which contain intrinsic histone acetyltransferase (HAT) activity. This allows subsequent local acetylation of histones, remodeling of the local DNA and RNA polymerase II-mediated gene transcription.[14] Reversal of this acetylation by histone deacetylases (HDACs) can reverse or block gene expression.

GR is a modular transcription factor with distinct regions associated with specific functions, such as ligand binding, nuclear translocation, and binding to

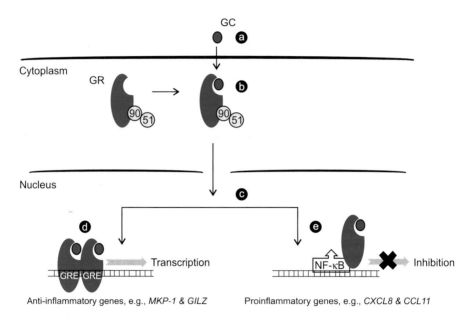

Figure 9-1 Mechanism of action of glucocorticoid steroid (GC). (a) The GC enters the cytoplasm, where (b) it binds to the cytosolic glucocorticoid receptor (GR) complex (including chaperone proteins Hsp90 and Hsp51). The GC/GR complex translocates into the nucleus (c) where it either binds the glucocorticoid responsive element (GRE) as a homodimer resulting in the upregulation of anti-inflammatory gene, such as mitogen activated protein kinase phosphatase (MKP)1 and glucocorticoid-inducible leucine zipper (GILZ), (d) or it acts to prevent proinflammatory transcription factors such as NF-κ(kappa)B from stimulating proinflammatory gene expression, e.g., that of CXCL8 and CCL11 (e).

transcriptional coactivator proteins or repressors.[14] The inability of CS to function effectively in refractory asthma has been linked to abnormalities at each stage of GR activation namely GR expression, ligand binding, nuclear translocation, and/or binding to GRE (Figure 9-1).[7-9,22]

Gene Induction by Corticosteroids

Activated GR acts as a transcription factor within the nucleus with a dual role. By recruiting distinct cofactor complexes, possibly under the control of posttranslational modifications, it can either enhance or suppress gene expression. Gene induction is associated with activated GR binding as a homodimer to a specific GREs within the promoter region of corticosteroid responsive genes. The 15bp consensus GRE is composed of an imperfect palindrome of 2 hexamers separated by a 3bp linker AGAACA*nnn*TGTTCT.[23] The majority of bases within a GRE can be modified without unduly affecting DNA binding *per se*.[24] However, as previously described for NF-κB sites,[25] even a single base pair change can affect the functional response either through alteration of the GR conformation on DNA and/or cofactor association.[26]

Moreover, in relation to gene induction, only the GRE flanking regions are conserved across cells and species in a gene specific manner. These flanking regions contain binding motifs for AP-1, ETS, SP1, C/EBP, and HNF2 transcription factors. Activated GR can interact with these DNA binding factors to provide a scaffold enabling gene specific combinatorial modulation of transcriptional responses.[24,27] In contrast to most transcription factors, analyzed to date, which bind to promoter regions just upstream to the transcription start site (TSS), only 17% of GREs are found close to and upstream from a TSS.[24,27] Furthermore, studies suggest that there are distinct differences in the positions of GR-DNA binding sites between genes that are activated and repressed. Thus, 234 genes are regulated by dexamethasone in A549 cells, and these are associated with 4392 distinct GR-DNA binding sites.[28] GR inducible genes had a median distance of GR-DNA binding 11 kb from the TSS, whereas repressed genes had a median distance of 146 kb. Furthermore, gene induction responses were more rapid than gene expression and interestingly, genes controlling circadian rhythm were regulated at low-concentrations of dexamethasone.[28]

This concept has changed the authors view for GR interaction with DNA.[26] The GRE is, in reality, a composite element which allows GR to perform distinct regulatory roles in a cell and context dependent manner. So, for example, the presence of activated GR in a complex may not modulate gene expression unless the correct profile of composite factors is present; DNA accessibility is achieved or cofactor recruitment complete.[29] Thus, we must consider DNA as a sequence specific allosteric ligand of GR that tailors the activity of the receptor toward specific target genes in much the same way that different CS ligands have subtle differences on GR function.[26] This together with the recent knowledge as to the regulation of GR gene induction by cofactor association by different phosphorylation events,[30,31] has greatly advanced our knowledge, of the complexity of gene induction by activated GR.

The activation status of p38 mitogen activated protein kinase (MAPK) and jun-N-terminal kinase (JNK) is controlled by the actions of phosphatases, including MAPK phosphatase 1 (MKP-1). MKP-1 induction is impaired in airway cells from patients with severe asthma and this may account, at least in part, for the elevated activation of p38 MAPK seen in severe asthma.[32-34] The mechanism by which dexamethasone switches on MKP-1 expression appears to be unique in that GR monomers, rather than dimers which binds to 3 distinct GRE half sites.[35]

Gene Repression by Corticosteroids

GR induced anti-inflammatory gene induction is important in controlling the inflammatory response, but activated GR can also suppress proinflammatory gene transcription. Activated GR can either directly bind to a GRE that sit across the TSS of inflammatory genes or indirectly through the inhibition of other transcription factors, such as AP-1 and NF-κB.[14]

NF-κB is maintained in the cytoplasm of the unstimulated cells by interaction with the inhibitor of NF-κB (IκB). Once the cell is stimulated by proinflammatory cytokines, such as TNF-α, IκB-α is rapidly phosphorylated and ubiquitinated before being degraded in the proteosome. This results in the release of active NF-κB heterodimers, which can then translocate into the nucleus. In the nucleus, NF-κB binds to gene promoters in responsive genes. In addition, it transcriptionally regulates IκB, resulting in a negative feedback loop as NF-κB is resequestered to the cytoplasm.[36] The interaction between GR and NF-κB is mutually antagonistic and activation of the NF-κB pathway can therefore result in repression of GR function.[37] Importantly, increased NF-κB activation is associated with severe asthma and chronic obstructive pulmonary disease (COPD).[16]

The interaction between NF-κB and GR is mutually antagonistic in that elevated GR blocks the actions of NF-κB and increased NF-κB attenuates GR functions and is controlled by the GR acetylation status.[37] Upon ligand binding, GR is rapidly acetylated at aa492-495; however, only the deacetylated form of GR is able to associate with the p65 subunit of NF-κB. Deacetylation of GR is controlled by HDAC2.[37] In addition to GR deacetylation, HDAC2 also reverses local histone acetylation (see later) and subsequent expression of CXCL8 and granulocyte macrophage colony-stimulating factor (GM-CSF).[37] HDAC2 expression and/or activity has been shown to be reduced in severe asthma patients, particularly children,[38] and this is more pronounced in patients with COPD.[39] Interestingly, GRβ has been reported to reduce HDAC2 expression in human bronchoalveolar lavage (BAL) macrophages.[40]

The role of HDAC2 in corticoid insensitivity is not limited to deacetylation of GR. The primary function of HDAC proteins is to alter the acetylation status of histone proteins. In the resting cell, chromatin is present in a highly compacted state which prevents transcription factor accessibility.[41] During activation of the cell, this compact inaccessible chromatin is made available to DNA binding proteins, thus, allowing the induction of gene transcription.[41] Since increased gene transcription is associated with increased HAT activity and local histone acetylation, loss of a specific HDAC may lead to changes in the chromatin structure at the promoter regions of inflammatory genes and thereby, altering transcription factor DNA binding, and subsequent gene expression.[42-45]

More recently, a novel type of repressive function of GR has been described whereby, GR binds to a palindromic sequencing consisting of 2 inverted repeats (IR) separated by a single bp (IR1 nGRE).[46] These sequences are implicated in the control of over 1000 genes in man.[46]

Type 2 T Helper Cell Mediators and Refractory Asthma

Binding of a ligand to GR within the cytoplasm leads to a conformational change in GR, its dissociation from the multisubunit Hsp90 complex and formation of a transcriptionally active form of GR.[14]

The binding affinity of a GR ligand binding can be reduced in T lymphocytes by certain cytokines, such as IL-2, IL-4, and IL-13, which are overexpressed in a subtype of refractory asthma patients.[16,20] Overexpression within the airways of these cytokines may cause a localized glucocorticoids (GC) resistance, possibly as a result of GRβ induction.[20] GR activity is regulated by posttranslational modifications, such as phosphorylation.[47] The activation of p38 MAPK by Th2 cytokines can result in GR phosphorylation at specific sites leading to reduced GR activity.[33] The activation domain of GR possess 5 known phosphorylation sites on serine residues S113, S141, S203, S211, and S226. Some of these sites (S203, S211, and S226) are phosphorylated in newly translated GR, but are removed immediately as GR becomes part of the multi-subunit Hsp90 complex. The phosphatases involved in GR dephosphorylation at specific sites requires elucidation. Dissociation of the Hsp90 complex upon GR ligand binding allows number of kinases to target GR, which becomes phosphorylated. GR phosphorylation status can alter GR function, for example, phosphorylation of Ser211 correlates with ligand binding, nuclear translocation, and transactivation.[47]

Precisely, how p38 MAPK regulates the inflammatory response and corticosteroid function in refractory asthma is an area of great interest.[7] p38 MAPK overexpression is associated with GC resistance to burn injury in mice[48] and p38 MAPK inhibitors were able to restore GC sensitivity in peripheral blood cells and BAL macrophages in patients with severe asthma.[33,49,50] The expression and activity of p38 MAPK is elevated in these patients without directly modulating the expression of inflammatory cytokines released from these cells.[33,49,50] The data indicate that a combination of a p38 MAPK inhibitor with an ICS, but neither alone, may be of clinical benefit. Interestingly, the activity of p38 MAPK is enhanced by p300-mediated acetylation.[51]

Intriguingly, Goleva et al. demonstrated that this effect of p38 MAPK inhibition in restoring GR function was mimicked by interferon (IFN-γ).[49] Other MAPKs, particularly the MEK/ERK pathway, have also been associated with reduced GC responsiveness in cells from patients with refractory asthma depending upon the precise cell activation protocol used refractory asthma.[52,53] In other kinases, such as cyclin dependent kinase (CDK), glycogen synthase kinase-3, and JNKs can also target the phosphorylation sites on GR.[7,9]

A number of phosphatases including PP1, PP2A and PP5 can regulate GR nuclear import and/or function possibly through alteration in GR phosphorylation status.[14] As for example, PP5 which is part of the Hsp90/GR complex can modulate GR phosphorylation and the subsequent expression of subsets of GR inducible genes in different cell types.[14] Furthermore, induction of PP5 by estrogen in breast cancer cell lines leads to dephosphorylation of GR and reduced functional responses.[54] Analysis of phosphatase expression and activity in primary cells from patients with severe asthma may reveal important differences.

Another mechanism by which p38 MAPK may regulate CS sensitivity in human T cells has also been described. In T cells, p38 MAPK mediated activation of GATA3 can also regulate GR nuclear import.[55]

There is often a divergent response to GCs between CD4+ and CD8+ T cells, resulting in lingering populations of CD8+ cells despite systemic GC treatment.[56,57] Although the mechanisms of GC actions are the same in both cell types, alternate effects of GC on histone acetylation has been observed.[57] The differences in histone H4 acetylation has been attributed to deficient HAT activity, specifically of ATF2, in the CD8+ cells, resulting in reduced gene silencing.[57]

Interleukin-17 and Type 17 T Helper Cells in Refractory Asthma

Th17 cells represent a distinct population of CD4+ Th cells that mediate neutrophilic inflammation and are characterized by the production of IL-17, IL-22, and IL-6 under the control of the Th17 selective transcription factor, related orphan receptor (ROR)γt.[58] IL-17 upregulates the expression of a number of CXCR2 chemokines including CXCL1, CXCL6, and CXCL8 together with neutrophil survival factors GM-CSF and G-CSF from the airway epithelium.[58] Adoptive transfer of polarized Th17 cells into ovalbumin challenged mice resulted in a dexamethasone insensitive predominantly neutrophilic inflammatory response and aryl hydrocarbon receptor (AHR) to metacholine.[59] IL-17 has also been reported to affect structural cells and to stimulate the production of profibrotic cytokines and extracellular matrix proteins.[58] In addition, IL-17 can act synergistically with viral infection or other inflammatory mediators including TNF-α to potentiate these responses.[58] These data clearly indicate the possibility that IL-17 and Th17 cells play a major role in severe asthma and several groups have analyzed IL-17 expression in various biological samples from patients with severe refractory asthma.

IL-17 levels in sputum[60] and serum[61] are elevated in severe asthma with sputum IL-17 correlating with neutrophilia.[60] In addition, serum IL-17 level >20 pg/mL is an independent risk factor for severe asthma.[61] Furthermore, using principal component analysis, one of the dominant variables for severe asthmatics with intermittent airflow obstruction was IL-17 along with IL-9, monocyte chemotactic protein 1, and RANTES.[62]

Although investigators reported increased IL-17A expression in infiltrating cells in severe asthma,[63] this was not confirmed in a more recent study.[64] Both groups did however, report increased IL-17F positive cells in the epithelium[63] and submucosa of severe asthmatics.[64] There was no evidence that IL-17A and IL-17F positive cells correlated directly with neutrophilic inflammation, but IL-17F positive cells correlated with the submucosal eosinophils.[64]

The proinflammatory function of IL-17A depends on IL-22 availability and increased IL-22 levels are found in the serum of patients with asthma. In IL-22 knockout mice eosinophil recruitment, Th2 cytokine production, mucus production, and airway hyper-reactivity are drastically reduced following ovalbumin challenge.[65]

Type 1 T Helper Cells in Refractory Asthma

The expression of many genes induced by IFN-γ, or the combination of IFN-γ and TNF-α, are relatively GC insensitive, despite the same genes being steroid sensitive when induced by other stimuli.[66] IFN-γ activates the transcription factor, IFN regulatory factor (IRF)-1, overexpression of which in human airway smooth muscle cells results in the abrogation of GR function[67] through competition for limiting amounts of the transcriptional coregulator GR-interacting protein 1 (GRIP-1).[68]

In human airway smooth muscle cells, GRIP-1 forms a coactivating complex with phosphorylated GR enabling the modulation of a distinct pattern of anti-inflammatory genes[68] as well as, in ligand and promoter specific transrepression.[69] In addition, GRIP-1 physically interacts with IRF-1 to enable the production of key inflammatory genes, such as RANTES and CD38.[68] IRF-1 can compete with GR for GRIP-1 resulting in attenuation of GR function, potentially playing a role in steroid insensitivity in severe asthma and COPD.[68] The expression of GRIP-1 in these diseases needs to be determined.

Chronic persistent obstruction in severe asthma is associated with earlier age of onset, longer disease duration, more inflammatory cells in the sputum, and greater smooth muscle area. Although, no biomarker distinguished chronic persistent from intermittent airflow obstruction, principal component analysis revealed that the dominant variables in the chronic persistent obstruction group were IL-12, IL-13, and IFN-γ.[62]

Regulatory T Cells

GCs induce the key anti-inflammatory gene, IL-10[14] in regulatory T cells (Treg) cells thereby inhibiting cytokine secretion by activated Th2 cells. Importantly, this induction is impaired in some Cheyne-Stokes respiration (CSR) patients.[70] Costimulation of these IL-10 producing deficient Treg cells with dexamethasone and vitamin D3 (calcitriol) *in vitro* restores IL-10 secretion back to levels seen in cells from GC-sensitive patients.[70] Furthermore, treatment of 3 CSR patients for several days with vitamin D3 restored *in vitro* Treg cell function with respect to IL-10 production, suggesting that this might be a useful therapeutic approach.[70] Therefore, low dietary intake of vitamin D or lack of sunlight might be contributory factors to reduced GC responses in inflammatory diseases. The results of clinical trials with vitamin D3 supplementation in patients, both adults and children, with refractory asthma are awaited.

Dendritic Cells

There is much recent interest in the role dendritic cells (DCs) and the inflammasome in modulating asthmatic inflammation.[71] DCs can sense the airway environment and are activated in asthma in response to allergic and noxious stimuli.[70] Activation of DCs in response to fungal infection for example can lead to the release of TNF-α and the subsequent induction of IL-17A and IL-5 within the lungs which in combination can enhance the expression of neutrophil chemoattractants. This combination results in an airway neutrophilia which overrides the classic asthmatic eosinophil response.[72] In the mouse, TNF-α may therefore be considered as a key mediator regulating DC and CD4 T cell interactions to promote neutrophilic airway inflammation.[71]

The release of innate immune mediators from bronchial epithelial cells can modulate the function of DCs which recognize and sample inhaled allergens. This, in turn, results in the initiation and maintenance of adaptive Th2 responses in asthma.[73] DC-derived chemokines, such as the CCR4 ligands, CCL17, and CCL22 attract Th2 cells to the airway in a humanized mouse model of HDM-induced AHR.[74] In addition, during Th2-mediated inflammation, DCs mature and this status is maintained even after resolution of Th2-mediated inflammatory response. These mature DCs facilitate a subsequent Th2 response to neoantigens.[75] This suggests that regulation of DC function may control the autoimmune response produced in response to oxidative stress mediated modification of self-proteins which leads to neoantigen formation.[76]

Recent data show elevated levels of uric acid following allergen challenge in asthmatics and in animal models of asthma.[77] In addition, uric acid, in the presence of an antigen, was able to induce an asthma-like phenotype in mice. The mechanism for this adjuvant effect of uric acid was via activation of DCs through spleen tyrosine kinase and PI3-kinase δ signalling. In contrast, no role for IL-1β or the NLRP3 inflammasome was seen.[77]

IL-1β is often present in Th17-driven inflammatory diseases. IL-1β secretion requires the action of caspase-1-dependent processing of pro-IL-1β following microbial and environmental stimulation of the NLRP3 inflammasome.[78] Indeed, elevated levels of IL-1β, IL-17, and the acute-phase protein serum amyloid A (SAA) are present in subjects with severe allergic asthma. SAA is also expressed in the lungs of mice exposed to different allergic sensitization regimens, which produce a mixed Th2/Th17 response and SAA instillation results in an IL-1-dependent lung neutrophilia. This effect is downstream of IL-1α, IL-1β, IL-6, and IL-23 production and DC maturation. NLRP3 inflammasome activation is required for IL-1β release from DCs and the subsequent stimulation of TNF-α production from CD4+ T cells.[79]

Superantigen

The pathology of intrinsic and extrinsic asthma is similar, indeed immunoglobulin E (IgE) synthesis has been found in the airways of intrinsic asthmatics despite negative skin prick tests and serum specific IgE.[80] Microbial superantigens, particularly staphylococcal enterotoxins are probably more important in amplifying inflammation in these patients rather than driving intrinsic asthma itself.[80] Super-antigens may be important in intrinsic asthma as airway epithelial cells may be colonized by staphylococci and other superantigen producing microbes leading to local production of specific IgE as well as polyclonal IgE. Specific IgE antibodies against staphylococcal enterotoxins have been found in patients with severe asthma and are able to sensitize mast cells and DCs.[80,81]

Superantigens cause mast cell activation, clonal expansion of T cells, and suppression of Treg cells. Cytotoxic autoantibodies may also be implicated as IgG antibodies directed against epithelial proteins, such as cytokeratin-18, which have been detected in intrinsic asthma.[80] In a small study investigating the link between asthma and autoimmune conditions, Agache et al. reported that the presence of antinuclear antigens (ANA) in severe asthmatics was associated with death, severe exacerbations, high ICS intake, and with an annual decline in forced expiratory volume in 1 second (FEV_1) >100 mL.[82] In addition, autoantibodies against α-enolase protein have been associated with severe asthma.[83,84] These antibodies were IgG1 in nature, which may be implicated in complement activation in these subjects. This may be particularly important in female patients with late-onset severe asthma.

Staphylococcal enterotoxin B can stimulate Th17 cells, which may be important in driving neutrophilic inflammation in more severe asthma.[85] Staphylococcal superantigens may also inhibit the immunosuppressive activity of Treg and may therefore amplify the activity of Th2 cells and CD8+ cells.[86] Staphylococcal enterotoxin B inhibits CD4+ CD25+ Tregs by inducing the protein GC-induced TNF receptor-related protein ligand (GITR) in monocytes.[87]

Superantigens have also been shown to induce CS resistance by activating the ERK/MAPK pathway either through increasing expression of GRβ or by affecting GRα phosphorylation status. In either case, CS responsiveness was restored by coincubation with a selective ERK inhibitor.[52] In addition, activation of DCs obtained from patients with systemic lupus erythematosus (SLE) through TLR7 and TLR9 can reduce the ability of dexamethasone to attenuate NF-κB activation and DC cell death and subsequent attenuation of IFN-α levels.[88]

Reactive Oxygen Species/Reactive Nitrogen Species

There is high level of oxidative stress in patients with refractory asthma compared to the control population and GR translocation has been shown to be reduced by oxidative stress.[89] Hydrogen peroxide (H_2O_2) *in vitro* reduces dexamethasone induced GR translocation in primary human airway fibroblasts.[89] Oxidative stress may, therefore, not only play a role in amplifying inflammation in severe refractory asthma and COPD, but may also be important as a modulator of CS action in smoking asthmatics and nonsmoking severe asthma patients.[90] Antioxidants may therefore improve GR nuclear translocation[8,9] and potentially be able to act in concert with the combination of ICS and LABA which together show significantly higher levels of GR nuclear translocation than ICS alone both *in vitro* and *in vivo*.[91]

AP-1 expression is greater in peripheral blood mononuclear cells (PBMCs) from CSR patients compared to those from steroid sensitive asthmatics (SSA).[92] AP-1 is comprised of variable heterodimers of Jun (c-Jun, Jun B, and Jun D) and Fos (c-Fos, Fos B, Fra-1 and Fra-2), although the most stable complex in activated cells is the c-Fos/c-Jun heterodimer.[93] AP-1 can drive the expression of several key asthma genes including *IL-5, GMCSF, TGF-β*, and *TNF-α*.[93] As with NF-κB, AP-1 can mutually repress GR functions and overexpression of AP-1 or enhanced JNK activity has been proposed as a mechanism of GC resistance in asthma.[14,94] Evidence suggests that JNK is activated and both c-fos and c-jun expression is enhanced to a greater extent in PBMCs and bronchial biopsies from patients with refractory asthma compared to nonsevere asthma. Furthermore, in PBMCs from patients with GC-resistant asthma, there is no reduction in JNK activity or c-Jun after high doses of oral GC.[7]

Excess production of reactive oxygen species (ROS) leads to the induction of nitric oxide (NO) synthase (NOS) and elevated levels of NO.[90] This may account for the enhanced localized production of NO which is found in patients with steroid refractory asthma.[95] NO reacts with critical sulhydryl (SH) groups on GR resulting in nitrosylation of GR or GR-associated protein and alterations of ligand binding and/or affinity.[7,96] However, this may be selective for specific GR residues as the NO donating steroid NCX-1080 can enhance GR function.[97] The effects of NO may be higher in smoking asthmatics, due to the conversion of NO to peroxynitrate, which can also induce steroid insensitivity.[90] Furthermore, nitrosylation of HDAC2 can attenuate its activity thereby potentially affecting GR function.[98] For this reason, treatment with NOS inhibitors and/or antioxidants may provide benefit for CSR patients.[7]

Oxidative and nitrosative stress result in the formation of peroxynitrite, which nitrates tyrosine residues on HDAC2 resulting in its inactivation, ubiquitination, and degradation.[99] More recently, S-nitrosylation of HDAC2 on Cys262 and Cys274 has been reported to affect its chromatin binding capacity and this may also contribute to reduced GR function.[98]

The suppression of lipopolysuccharide (LPS)-induced cytokine release (CCL2, CCL3, CCL5, TNF-α, IL-1β, CXCL8, IFN-γ, IL-6, IL-10, and GM-CSF) by dexamethasone from PBMCs of CSR patients was reduced compared to that seen in mild SSA.[100] Nuclear HDAC and HAT activities were reduced in patients with CSR compared with patients with SSA and, importantly, the reduced HDAC activity correlated directly with steroid insensitivity. In contrast, the reduction in

HAT activity related to corticosteroid use rather than asthma severity.[100] Similar results have been reported in children where severity of disease was measured by bronchial hyper-responsiveness.[38]

However, reduced HDAC2 expression has not been seen in all CSR patients reflecting the heterogeneity of severe asthma phenotype and the possible role of other HDACs in GR function.[101] HDAC2 has been shown to be important in GR-mediated repression of inflammatory genes, such as GM-CSF and CXCL8,[37] and its expression and activity is decreased in smokers, smoking asthmatics, COPD,[102] and in cystic fibrosis,[103] all of which are known to be insensitive to the anti-inflammatory effects of GCs. Furthermore, the repressive effect of dexamethasone on CXCL8 and TNF production is negatively correlated with total HDAC activity in alveolar macrophages from smokers and nonsmokers.[104]

Overexpression of HDAC2, but not HDAC1, in primary macrophages from COPD patients restored dexamethasone efficacy towards suppressing LPS-induced GM-CSF release to levels seen in cells from healthy control subjects.[37] Furthermore, knockdown of HDAC2 in sputum macrophages from healthy nonsmokers by RNAi reduced the inhibitory effect of dexamethasone.[37] Recent evidence suggests that there is a link between GRβ and HDAC2 in patients with severe steroid insensitive asthma.[40] Thus, increased GRβ expression selectively reduces HDAC2 and can prevent GRα-induced enhancement of HDAC2 promoter reporter gene activity in a concentration dependent manner. Treatment options for the restoration of HDAC2 may include the bronchodilator theophylline, which has been used *in vitro* to restore HDAC2 activity independent of its actions on PDE4[102] and in COPD patients.[105] Theophylline at subbronchodilator doses may, therefore, have potential in restoring GC sensitivity at least in smoking asthmatics.[102]

Oxidative stress also activates phosphoinositide-3-kinase (PI3K)-δ, which leads to phosphorylation and inactivation of HDAC2.[106,107] The authors demonstrated in both animal models and in *ex vivo* studies that pharmacological or genetic inhibition of PI3Kδ, but not PI3Kγ, enhanced steroid responsiveness.[106,107]

Other HDACs have also been implicated in the regulation GR function. There are 18 HDACs in total belonging to 4 major classes[108] and the precise role for each individual enzyme in lung disease requires further investigation. HDAC6 reversibly acetylates the GR chaperone Hsp90 which can affect the release and maturation of the activated GR complex and attenuation of GR nuclear translocation.[109,110] Dexamethasone-induced repression of Th2 cytokines required GR to bring HDAC1 to GATA3 located on the promoters of Th2 genes.[111] HDAC3 can also modulate GR functions: HDAC3 complexes with silencing mediator for retinoid and thyroid receptors (SMRT) and nuclear receptor corepressor (N-CoR) to obtain full activity and is recruited to GR repressing its transactivation function by the action of the chaperone protein Bcl-2 associated athanogene 1M (Bag-1M).[112] Recently, SIRT1 (a member of the sirtuin family of deacetylases) has been reported to act as a major repressor of dexamethasone-induced uncoupling protein-3 (UCP3) expression through deacetylation of the *ucp3* promoter. This effect is indirect through impairing the association of p300 with GR.[113] Histone methyltransferases have also been reported to play a role in GR function.[114]

Genetic Factors

The extent to which refractory asthma is caused by specific genetic events is still under debate. Asthma heritability estimates vary from 40 to 60%, and it was predicted that genome-wide association studies (GWAS), which permit the analysis of hundreds of thousands of gene polymorphisms from thousands of individuals at reasonable cost and speed in an hypothesis-independent fashion would be helpful in identifying genes involved in the pathophysiology of the disease and in identifying new therapeutic targets.[115,116] There have now been over 670 genes associated with asthma (the Human Genetic Epidemiology Navigator database)[116] and GWAS results have generated novel disease loci albeit of modest effects whilst supporting previous studies in distinct populations.[115,117] However, only a small fraction of heritability can be explained by the major susceptibility single nucleotide polymorphism (SNPs) identified in most complex diseases.[118] In asthma, the major susceptibility loci detected by GWAS are linked to genes that have not previously been associated with disease. The evidence from GWAS suggests genetic differences between childhood and adult onset asthma in Caucasians and a distinct pattern of hits in other ethnic groups particularly those of African ancestry.[118] Asthma is a heterogeneous disease/syndrome[119] and data from the National Institutes of Health (NIH) Severe Asthma Research programme (SARP) indicate that asthma clusters into distinct cohorts that are independent of ethnic background in adults,[3] but not children.[120]

The first GWAS in asthma reported global significance for SNPs located at chromosome 17q21 close to the genes for ORMDL3 and GSDMB,[121] and this was confirmed in a larger study.[122] Other genes, such as IL1RL1/IL18R1, HLA-DQ, IL-33, SMAD3, and IL2RB were also implicated in asthma in this study.[122] The association of ORMDL3 with asthma has been replicated in diverse populations by GWAS except for those of African ancestry.[117] The clinical relevance of ORMDL3 in asthma *per se* remains unclear although a link with altered SERCA activity has been proposed.[123]

PBMCs from healthy subjects treated with GCs indicate that nearly 25% exhibit some form of resistance to dexamethasone.[124] The data indicate that a proportion of the general population who have an attenuated GC sensitivity which would only become manifest if the subject developed a disease requiring GC therapy.[22] Furthermore, alterations in specific genes, such as the p50 component of NF-κB and the GR chaperone protein FKBP51 have been proposed to play a role in CSR, but this link is still unproven.[22]

A missense mutation of GR can cause global insensitivity to steroid actions.[125] GC insensitivity syndrome was first described in 1976[126] in patients with hyper-cortisolism without Cushingoid features. This is a very rare genetic disease with >20 kindreds and occasional sporadic cases due to GR mutations. This leads to elevated circulating cortisol levels due to a resetting of the hypothalamic preoptic adrenal (HPA) axis.[127] The disease presents with a broad clinical spectrum from completely asymptomatic to mild and to severe symptomatic conditions. Indeed, most subjects are asymptomatic with only biochemical changes being apparent.[127] Although, most of the sequence changes result in a loss of GR function, some mutations, such as N363S, are linked to increased GR function.[128] GR mutations result in a number of defects in GR function including decreases in GR number, ligand binding, stability, nuclear translocation, and coactivator interaction leading to alterations in GR transactivation and transrepression.[127] For example, GR nuclear translocation is reduced with the I559N mutant resulting in attenuation of GRE-mediated gene transduction.[129]

CLINICAL IMPLICATIONS

Unbiased cluster analysis of patients with severe asthma may in future reveal key changes in the inflammatory profile or specific pathways that are aberrantly activated in these patients, which could lead to the development of novel treatments in the future.[130] However, it is clear that relative GC insensitive patients who are smokers should be encouraged to quit to prevent the redox drive.[90] Clinical data indicate the subsets of patients with steroid-refractory asthma will respond to specific anti-inflammatory agents, e.g., anti-IL-5.[131,132] Other drugs directed against Th2 cytokines, e.g., IL-4 and IL-13 may also be of benefit in distinct patient subsets.[8,133] The single mediator approach, however, has not proved as successful as anticipated in small clinical trials in severe asthma even when specific subsets of patients are examined. Newer more general anti-inflammatory approached may, therefore, be necessary.[8,134]

In contrast to the development of a novel anti-inflammatory agent, it may be possible through the greater understanding of the pathways and mediators that prevent GC function in severe asthma to develop a drug that can restore the functional effects of ICS independent of the intrinsic anti-inflammatory efficacy of the drug (Figure 9-2). As described above, a number of key pathways and mediators have been implicated in controlling GC function which have proved abnormal in cells from severe asthmatics (Table 9-1).

For example, alterations in GR or GR cofactor phosphorylation can markedly attenuate GC function and modulation of p38 MAPK or PI3Kδ pathways may be one approach to restore steroid responsiveness. There may also be benefits in relation to side effects in that the novel compounds will be steroid sparing and the steroid

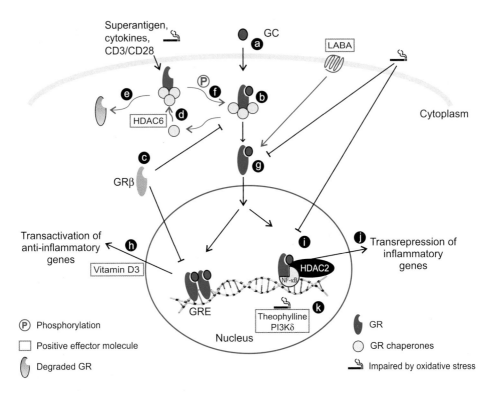

Figure 9-2 Mechanism of glucocorticoid steroid (GC) action by the glucocorticoid receptor (GR) and sites of regulation in GC insensitivity. The GC enters the cytoplasm by diffusion across the cell membrane (a), where it binds (b) to the GR. The increased expression of the GRβ isoform found in some patients with GC insensitive severe asthma can act as a dominant negative regulator of GRα (c). Ligand binding induces the release of chaperones proteins including Hsp90 (d), which is deacetylated by histone deacetylase (HDAC)6 enabling binding to immature GR. Cytoplasmic GR can be targeted for protease degradation by oxidative stress, which is increased in smokers and asthmatics (e) or phosphorylated by p38 mitogen activated protein kinase (MAPK) or other MAPKs and inactivated (f). In a similar manner, superantigen T-cell receptor costimulation (CD3/CD28) and enhanced expression of cytokines, such as interleukin (IL)-2 and IL-4 can lead to GR phosphorylation via MAPK pathways. Active GR translocates to the nucleus (g), which can be inhibited by oxidative stress, superantigen and inflammatory mediators or enhanced by long acting β-agonists (LABAs). GR homodimers can bind to the glucocorticoid response element (GRE) in anti-inflammatory genes, such as IL-10 inducing their expression (h). Impaired transactivation can be restored by vitamin D3 in a subset of SCR patients. GR can also interact with other transcription factors, such as NF-κB or AP-1 (i) by a tethering mechanism to transrepress inflammatory genes (j). HDAC2 is essential for this process and can be reduced by oxidative stress, GRβ or enhanced expression of IL-2 and IL-4. HDAC2 is also important for deacetylation of core histones (k) resulting in tighter DNA packaging making inflammatory genes inaccessible to the transcriptional machinery. Again this can be reduced by oxidative stress and enhanced by drugs, such as theophylline which target PI3Kδ.

Table 9-1	Mediators and Pathways Implicated in Modulating Glucocorticoid Receptor Function
Mediators	*Signaling pathways*
• IL-2, IL-4[13,17] • IFNγ[23,48-50] • Oxidative stress[31] • Infection/TLR agonists[25,91,92,95] • Vitamin D3[42]	• Redox sensitive transcription factors, e.g., NF-κB[13,36,44,46,47] • PI3 kinase[56,57] • MAPK pathways (p38, JNK, ERK/MEK)[21-24,32] • GSK3β[9,46] • IRF-1[50] • CDK1[7] • Phosphatases PP1, PP2A, PP5[12,27] • HDAC2[44,52-60,63,64,67,71,79,80]

CDK, cyclin-dependent kinase; ERK, extracellular regulated kinase; HDAC, histone deacetylase; IFN, interferon; IL, interleukin; IRF, interferon regulatory factor; JNK, c-Jun N-terminal kinase; MAPK, mitogen-activated protein kinase; MEK, mitogen-activated protein kinase/extracellular signal-regulated kinase kinase; NF-κB, nuclear factor κB; PI3K, phosphoinositide-3-kinase; PP, protein phosphatase; TLR, toll-like receptor.

could also reduce potential side effects of the novel compound. In an open-label study in patients with steroid-refractory inflammatory bowel disease on high-dose oral steroids, addition of anti-IL-2 treatment proved of benefit.[124] Controlled studies using anti-IL-2 in severe asthma may, therefore, possibly be of benefit. The development of good noninvasive biomarkers of aberrant inflammatory pathway/ mediator activation and defective GR activation steps in severe asthma is essential for future patient directed approaches to work.

Asthma exacerbations, whether driven by bacterial infection, viruses or both, are relatively steroid insensitive, and may reflect an action of these infectious agents on GR function. Prolonged exposure of monocytes to LPS can induce a relative steroid insensitivity and importantly, LPS levels in BAL are raised in patients with severe asthma.[135] In a similar effect is seen with exposure of cells to superantigen[52] where this causes reduced GR nuclear import controlled by the MEK/ERK pathway.[52] Rhinoviral infection can also attenuate GR nuclear translocation and suppression of inflammatory cytokine release from primary human epithelial cells in an NF-κB dependent manner.[136] This indicates that anti-infective agents may be beneficial in severe asthma.

There is increasing evidence for an autoimmune component in asthma.[137] Many of the autoimmune diseases, such as SLE are relatively steroid insensitive and understanding how GR function is modulated by autoimmune mechanisms may provide further insight into treatment of these patients.[88] Stimulation of toll-like receptors (TLR)7 and TLR9 on DCs by self DNA can attenuate the ability of steroids to suppress NF-κB mediated IFN-α production *in vitro* and *in vivo*.[88] This suggests that TLR7 and/or TLR9 antagonists could be effective steroid sparing agents in the clinic.

ICS, with or without LABAs, are the mainstay of anti-inflammatory therapy for asthma. However, a significant percentage of subjects are refractory to their anti-inflammatory effects. The mechanisms underlying this refractoriness are being elucidated and appear to be patient and stimulus dependent with environmental factors playing an increasingly important role. Defining the abnormalities in signalling pathways or mediator expression that modulate GR function in severe asthma may result in new therapies for these subjects: either monotherapies or more likely novel combinations of ICS and kinase inhibitors. Changes in the epigenetic profile of key resident cells within the airways of severe asthmatics highlights the increasing awareness of how the environment, through epigenetics, can affect asthma susceptibility, development and severity, and possibly steroid functions. Restoration of the normal epigenetic profile to these abnormal structural cells from patients with severe asthma may potentially cure asthma and provides a new area for drug discovery.

CONCLUSION

Relative corticosteroid resistance has been a major area of research interest in asthma for over 40 years. The failure to respond to gold standard anti-inflammatory agents is associated with worse clinical outcomes and excessive healthcare cost. This highlights the need to understand the mechanisms that drive this relative corticosteroid resistance. Recent cluster analysis of clinical features has indicated that asthma is not a single disease but a syndrome in which numerous possibly overlapping clinical phenotypes occur. One of these phenotypes is corticosteroid resistance, which occurs in 5–10% of asthmatics. Within this phenotype, there is a potential to subclassify patients according to potential drivers for their steroid resistance, e.g., genetic susceptibility/family background, an excessive inflammatory drive which activates several distinct intracellular signalling pathways or cell activation by environmental stimuli such as pollution, cigarette smoke, and infections. Those asthmatics who smoke have reduced corticosteroid sensitivity and should undertake smoking cessation plans to reduce their oxidant and inflammatory load; and can potentially recover corticosteroid responsiveness. Despite marked advances in authors' knowledge of the diverse molecular and immune pathways that are implicated in asthma pathophysiology, novel therapies have either proved to have limited efficacy or are difficult to reach the market. Greater understanding of inflammatory signalling pathways that are abnormally activated in patients with severe corticosteroid-refractory asthma may lead to new anti-inflammatory approaches. Alternatively, appreciation of key pathways that modulate corticosteroid function may be targeted to overcome their relative corticosteroid resistance. The key to future treatments will be the development of noninvasive biomarkers for aberrant pathway activation if these specific approaches are to be successful. In the mid-term, conventional combination therapies will continue to be used but the addition of add-on treatments directed against aberrantly expressed inflammatory pathways or mediators are likely to prove the most effective therapies.

Acknowledgments

Research in the author's laboratories is supported by the EU (IMI), MRC (UK), Wellcome Trust, BBSRC, NERC, Asthma UK and by the NIH (USA). The authors have no conflicts of interest. The authors are principal investigators in the MRC/Asthma UK Centre for Asthma and Allergic Mechanisms.

REFERENCES

1. Holgate ST, Arshad HS, Roberts GC, Howarth PH, Thurner P, Davies DE. A new look at the pathogenesis of asthma. *Clin Sci* (*Lond*). 2009;118:439-50.
2. Haldar P, Pavord ID, Shaw DE, Berry MA, Thomas M, Brightling CE, et al. Cluster analysis and clinical asthma phenotypes. *Am J Respir Crit Care Med.* 2008;178:218-24.
3. Moore WC, Meyers DA, Wenzel SE, Teague WG, Li H, Li X, et al. Identification of asthma phenotypes using cluster analysis in the Severe Asthma Research Program. *Am J Respir Crit Care Med.* 2010;181:315-23.
4. Woodruff PG, Boushey HA, Dolganov GM, Barker CS, Yang YH, Donnelly S, et al. Genome-wide profiling identifies epithelial cell genes associated with asthma and with treatment response to corticosteroids. *Proc Natl Acad Sci U S A.* 2007;104:15858-63.
5. Barnes PJ. Inhaled glucocorticoids for asthma. *N Engl J Med.* 1995;332:868-75.
6. Chung KF, Caramori G, Adcock IM. Inhaled corticosteroids as combination therapy with beta-adrenergic agonists in airways disease: present and future. *Eur J Clin Pharmacol.* 2009;65:853-71.
7. Adcock IM, Barnes PJ. Molecular mechanisms of corticosteroid resistance. *Chest.* 2008; 134:394-401.
8. Adcock IM, Caramori G, Chung KF. New targets for drug development in asthma. *Lancet.* 2008;372:1073-87.
9. Barnes PJ, Adcock IM. Glucocorticoid resistance in inflammatory diseases. *Lancet.* 2009; 373:1905-17.
10. Chung KF, Godard P, Adelroth E, Ayres J, Barnes N, Barnes P, et al. Difficult/therapy-resistant asthma. The need for an integrated approach to define clinical phenotypes, evaluate risk factors, understand pathophysiology and find novel therapies. ERS Task Force on Difficult/Therapy-Resistant Asthma. European Respiratory Society. *Eur Respir J.* 1999;13:1198-208.
11. Proceedings of the ATS workshop on refractory asthma: current understanding, recommendations, and unanswered questions. American Thoracic Society. *Am J Respir Crit Care Med.* 2000;162:2341-51.
12. Barnes PJ. New therapies for asthma: is there any progress? *Trends Pharmacol Sci.* 2010;31:335-43.
13. Adcock IM, Maneechotesuwan K, Usmani O. Molecular interactions between glucocorticoids and long-acting beta2-agonists. *J Allergy Clin Immunol.* 2002;110:S261-8.
14. Beck IM, Vanden Berghe W, Vermeulen L, Yamamoto KR, Haegeman G, De Bosscher K. Crosstalk in inflammation: the interplay of glucocorticoid receptor-based mechanisms and kinases and phosphatases. *Endocr Rev.* 2009;30:830-82.

15. Adcock IM, Gilbey T, Gelder CM, Chung KF, Barnes PJ. Glucocorticoid receptor localization in normal and asthmatic lung. *Am J Respir Crit Care Med.* 1996;154:771-82.

16. Ito K, Chung KF, Adcock IM. Update on glucocorticoid action and resistance. *J Allergy Clin Immunol.* 2006;117:522-43.

17. Lu NZ, Cidlowski JA. Glucocorticoid receptor isoforms generate transcription specificity. *Trends Cell Biol.* 2006;16:301-7.

18. Zhou J, Cidlowski JA. The human glucocorticoid receptor: one gene, multiple proteins and diverse responses. *Steroids.* 2005;70:407-17.

19. Lewis-Tuffin LJ, Cidlowski JA. The physiology of human glucocorticoid receptor beta (hGRbeta) and glucocorticoid resistance. *Ann N Y Acad Sci.* 2006;1069:1-9.

20. Kino T, Su YA, Chrousos GP. Human glucocorticoid receptor isoform beta: recent understanding of its potential implications in physiology and pathophysiology. *Cell Mol Life Sci.* 2009;66:3435-48.

21. Rhen T, Cidlowski JA. Antiinflammatory action of glucocorticoids—new mechanisms for old drugs. *N Engl J Med.* 2005;353:1711-23.

22. Hew M, Chung KF. Corticosteroid insensitivity in severe asthma: significance, mechanisms and aetiology. *Intern Med J.* 2010;40:323-34.

23. Adcock IM, Caramori G. Cross-talk between pro-inflammatory transcription factors and glucocorticoids. *Immunol Cell Biol.* 2001;79:376-84.

24. So AY, Chaivorapol C, Bolton EC, Li H, Yamamoto KR. Determinants of cell- and gene-specific transcriptional regulation by the glucocorticoid receptor. *PLoS Genet.* 2007;3:e94.

25. Leung TH, Hoffmann A, Baltimore D. One nucleotide in a kappaB site can determine cofactor specificity for NF-kappaB dimers. *Cell.* 2004;118:453-64.

26. Meijsing SH, Pufall MA, So AY, Bates DL, Chen L, Yamamoto KR. DNA binding site sequence directs glucocorticoid receptor structure and activity. *Science.* 2009;324:407-10.

27. So AY, Cooper SB, Feldman BJ, Manuchehri M, Yamamoto KR. Conservation analysis predicts in vivo occupancy of glucocorticoid receptor-binding sequences at gluco-corticoid-induced genes. *Proc Natl Acad Sci U S A.* 2008;105:5745-9.

28. Reddy TE, Pauli F, Sprouse RO, Neff NF, Newberry KM, Garabedian MJ, et al. Genomic determination of the glucocorticoid response reveals unexpected mechanisms of gene regulation. *Genome Res.* 2009;19:2163-71.

29. Luecke HF, Yamamoto KR. The glucocorticoid receptor blocks P-TEFb recruitment by NFkappaB to effect promoter-specific transcriptional repression. *Genes Dev.* 2005; 19:1116-27.

30. Avenant C, Ronacher K, Stubsrud E, Louw A, Hapgood JP. Role of ligand-dependent GR phosphorylation and half-life in determination of ligand-specific transcriptional activity. *Mol Cell Endocrinol.* 2010;327:72-88.

31. Avenant C, Kotitschke A, Hapgood JP. Glucocorticoid receptor phosphorylation modu-lates transcription efficacy through GRIP-1 recruitment. *Biochemistry.* 2010;49: 972-85.

32. Bhavsar P, Hew M, Khorasani N, Torrego A, Barnes PJ, Adcock I, et al. Relative cortico-steroid insensitivity of alveolar macrophages in severe asthma compared to non-severe asthma. *Thorax.* 2008;63:784-90.

33. Bhavsar P, Khorasani N, Hew M, Johnson M, Chung KF. Effect of p38 MAPK inhibition on corticosteroid suppression of cytokine release in severe asthma. *Eur Respir J.* 2010; 35:750-6.

34. Clark AR, Martins JR, Tchen CR. Role of dual specificity phosphatases in biological responses to glucocorticoids. *J Biol Chem.* 2008;283:25765-9.

35. Tchen CR, Martins JR, Paktiawal N, Perelli R, Saklatvala J, Clark AR. Glucocorticoid regulation of mouse and human dual specificity phosphatase 1 (DUSP1) genes: unusual cis-acting elements and unexpected evolutionary divergence. *J Biol Chem*. 2010;285: 2642-52.

36. Perkins ND. Integrating cell-signalling pathways with NF-kappaB and IKK function. *Nat Rev Mol Cell Biol*. 2007;8:49-62.

37. Ito K, Yamamura S, Essilfie-Quaye S, Cosio B, Ito M, Barnes PJ, et al. Histone deacetylase 2-mediated deacetylation of the glucocorticoid receptor enables NF-kappaB suppression. *J Exp Med*. 2006;203:7-13.

38. Su RC, Becker AB, Kozyrskyj AL, Hayglass KT. Altered epigenetic regulation and increasing severity of bronchial hyperresponsiveness in atopic asthmatic children. *J Allergy Clin Immunol*. 2009;124:1116-8.

39. Ito K, Ito M, Elliott WM, Cosio B, Caramori G, Kon OM, et al. Decreased histone deacetylase activity in chronic obstructive pulmonary disease. *N Engl J Med*. 2005;352:1967-76.

40. Li LB, Leung DY, Martin RJ, Goleva E. Inhibition of histone deacetylase 2 expression by elevated glucocorticoid receptor beta in steroid-resistant asthma. *Am J Respir Crit Care Med*. 2010;182:877-83.

41. Li B, Carey M, Workman JL. The role of chromatin during transcription. *Cell*. 2007;128: 707-19.

42. Heintzman ND, Hon GC, Hawkins RD, Kheradpour P, Stark A, Harp LF, et al. Histone modifications at human enhancers reflect global cell-type-specific gene expression. *Nature*. 2009;459:108-12.

43. Roh TY, Cuddapah S, Cui K, Zhao K. The genomic landscape of histone modifications in human T cells. *Proc Natl Acad Sci USA*. 2006;103:15782-7.

44. Wang Z, Zang C, Rosenfeld JA, Schones DE, Barski A, Cuddapah S, et al. Combinatorial patterns of histone acetylations and methylations in the human genome. *Nat Genet*. 2008;40:897-903.

45. Wang Z, Zang C, Cui K, Schones DE, Barski A, Peng W, et al. Genome-wide mapping of HATs and HDACs reveals distinct functions in active and inactive genes. *Cell*. 2009; 138:1019-31.

46. Surjit M, Ganti KP, Mukherji A, Ye T, Hua G, Metzger D, et al. Widespread negative response elements mediate direct repression by agonist-liganded glucocorticoid receptor. *Cell*. 2011;145:224-41.

47. Weigel NL, Moore NL. Steroid receptor phosphorylation: a key modulator of multiple receptor functions. *Mol Endocrinol*. 2007;21:2311-9.

48. D'Elia M, Patenaude J, Dupras C, Bernier J. T cells from burn-injured mice demonstrate a loss of sensitivity to glucocorticoids. *Am J Physiol Endocrinol Metab*. 2010;299:E299-307.

49. Goleva E, Li LB, Leung DY. IFN-gamma reverses IL-2- and IL-4-mediated T-cell steroid resistance. *Am J Respir Cell Mol Biol*. 2009;40:223-30.

50. Kent LM, Smyth LJ, Plumb J, Clayton CL, Fox SM, Ray DW, et al. Inhibition of lipopolysaccharide-stimulated chronic obstructive pulmonary disease macrophage inflammatory gene expression by dexamethasone and the p38 mitogen-activated protein kinase inhibitor N-cyano-N'-(2-{[8-(2,6-difluorophenyl)-4-(4-fluoro-2-methylphenyl)-7-oxo-7,8-dihy dropyrido[2,3-d] pyrimidin-2-yl]amino}ethyl)guanidine (SB706504). *J Pharmacol Exp Ther*. 2009;328:458-68.

51. Pillai VB, Sundaresan NR, Samant SA, Wolfgeher D, Trivedi CM, Gupta MP. Acetylation of a conserved lysine residue in the ATP binding pocket of p38 augments its kinase activity during hypertrophy of cardiomyocytes. *Mol Cell Biol*. 2011;31:2349-63.

52. Li LB, Goleva E, Hall CF, Ou LS, Leung DY. Superantigen-induced corticosteroid resistance of human T cells occurs through activation of the mitogen-activated protein kinase kinase/extracellular signal-regulated kinase (MEK-ERK) pathway. *J Allergy Clin Immunol.* 2004;114:1059-69.

53. Tsitoura DC, Rothman PB. Enhancement of MEK/ERK signaling promotes glucocorticoid resistance in CD4+ T cells. *J Clin Invest.* 2004;113:619-27.

54. Zhang Y, Leung DY, Nordeen SK, Goleva E. Estrogen inhibits glucocorticoid action via protein phosphatase 5 (PP5)-mediated glucocorticoid receptor dephosphorylation. *J Biol Chem.* 2009;284:24542-52.

55. Maneechotesuwan K, Yao X, Ito K, Jazrawi E, Usmani OS, Adcock IM, et al. Suppression of GATA-3 nuclear import and phosphorylation: a novel mechanism of corticosteroid action in allergic disease. *PLoS Med.* 2009;6:e1000076.

56. Chrousos GP, Kino T. Intracellular glucocorticoid signaling: a formerly simple system turns stochastic. *Sci STKE.* 2005;2005:pe48.

57. Li LB, Leung DY, Strand MJ, Goleva E. ATF2 impairs glucocorticoid receptor-mediated transactivation in human CD8+ T cells. *Blood.* 2007;110:1570-7.

58. Traves SL, Donnelly LE. Th17 cells in airway diseases. *Curr Mol Med.* 2008;8:416-26.

59. McKinley L, Alcorn JF, Peterson A, Dupont RB, Kapadia S, Logar A, et al. TH17 cells mediate steroid-resistant airway inflammation and airway hyperresponsiveness in mice. *J Immunol.* 2008;181:4089-97.

60. Sun YC, Zhou QT, Yao WZ. Sputum interleukin-17 is increased and associated with airway neutrophilia in patients with severe asthma. *Chin Med J (Engl).* 2005;118:953-6.

61. Agache I, Ciobanu C, Agache C, Anghel M. Increased serum IL-17 is an independent risk factor for severe asthma. *Respir Med.* 2010;104:1131-7.

62. Kaminska M, Foley S, Maghni K, Storness-Bliss C, Coxson H, Ghezzo H, et al. Airway remodeling in subjects with severe asthma with or without chronic persistent airflow obstruction. *J Allergy Clin Immunol.* 2009;124:45-51.e1-4.

63. Al-Ramli W, Préfontaine D, Chouiali F, Martin JG, Olivenstein R, Lemière C, et al. T(H)17-associated cytokines (IL-17A and IL-17F) in severe asthma. *J Allergy Clin Immunol.* 2009; 123:1185-7.

64. Doe C, Bafadhel M, Siddiqui S, Desai D, Mistry V, Rugman P, et al. Expression of the T helper 17-associated cytokines IL-17A and IL-17F in asthma and COPD. *Chest.* 2010; 138:1140-7.

65. Besnard AG, Sabat R, Dumoutier L, Renauld JC, Willart M, Lambrecht B, et al. Dual Role of IL-22 in allergic airway inflammation and its cross-talk with IL-17A. *Am J Respir Crit Care Med.* 2011;183:1153-63.

66. Tudhope SJ, Catley MC, Fenwick PS, Russell REK, Rumsey WL, Newton R, et al. The role of IkappaB kinase 2, but not activation of NF-kappaB, in the release of CXCR3 ligands from IFNgamma-stimulated human bronchial epithelial cells. *J Immunol.* 2007;179:6237-45.

67. Tliba O, Damera G, Banerjee A, Gu S, Baidouri H, Keslacy S, et al. Cytokines induce an early steroid resistance in airway smooth muscle cells: novel role of interferon regulatory factor-1. *Am J Respir Cell Mol Biol.* 2008;38:463-72.

68. Bhandare R, Damera G, Banerjee A, Flammer JR, Keslacy S, Rogatsky I, et al. Glucocorticoid receptor interacting protein-1 restores glucocorticoid responsiveness in steroid-resistant airway structural cells. *Am J Respir Cell Mol Biol.* 2010;42:9-15.

69. Ronacher K, Hadley K, Avenant C, Stubsrud E, Simons SS Jr, Louw A, et al. Ligand-selective transactivation and transrepression via the glucocorticoid receptor: role of cofactor interaction. *Mol Cell Endocrinol.* 2009;299:219-31.

70. Xystrakis E, Kusumakar S, Boswell S, Peek E, Urry Z, Richards DF, et al. Reversing the defective induction of IL-10-secreting regulatory T cells in glucocorticoid-resistant asthma patients. *J Clin Invest*. 2006;116:146-55.

71. Lambrecht BN, Hammad H. The role of dendritic and epithelial cells as master regulators of allergic airway inflammation. *Lancet*. 2010;376:835-43.

72. Fei M, Bhatia S, Oriss TB, Yarlagadda M, Khare A, Akira S, et al. TNF-alpha from inflammatory dendritic cells (DCs) regulates lung IL-17A/IL-5 levels and neutrophilia versus eosinophilia during persistent fungal infection. *Proc Natl Acad Sci U S A*. 2011; 108:5360-5.

73. Hammad H, Lambrecht BN. Dendritic cells and airway epithelial cells at the interface between innate and adaptive immune responses. *Allergy*. 2011;66:579-87.

74. Perros F, Hoogsteden HC, Coyle AJ, Lambrecht BN, Hammad H. Blockade of CCR4 in a humanized model of asthma reveals a critical role for DC-derived CCL17 and CCL22 in attracting Th2 cells and inducing airway inflammation. *Allergy*. 2009;64:995-1002.

75. van Rijt LS, Vos N, Willart M, Muskens F, Tak PP, van der Horst C, et al. Persistent activation of dendritic cells after resolution of allergic airway inflammation breaks tolerance to inhaled allergens in mice. *Am J Respir Crit Care Med*. 2011;184:303-11.

76. Kirkham PA, Caramori G, Casolari P, Papi A, Edwards M, Shamji B, et al. Oxidative Stress-induced Antibodies to Carbonyl-modified Protein Correlate with Severity of COPD.

77. Kool M, Willart MA, van Nimwegen M, Bergen I, Pouliot P, Virchow JC, et al. An unexpected role for uric acid as an inducer of T helper 2 cell immunity to inhaled antigens and inflammatory mediator of allergic asthma. *Immunity*. 2011;34:527-40.

78. Martinon F, Mayor A, Tschopp J. The inflammasomes: guardians of the body. *Annu Rev Immunol*. 2009;27:229-65.

79. Ather JL, Ckless K, Martin R, Foley KL, Suratt BT, Boyson JE, et al. Serum amyloid A activates the NLRP3 inflammasome and promotes Th17 allergic asthma in mice. *J Immunol*. 2011;187:64-73.

80. Barnes PJ. Intrinsic asthma: not so different from allergic asthma but driven by superantigens? *Clin Exp Allergy*. 2009;39:1145-51.

81. Gould HJ, Takhar P, Harries HE, Chevretton E, Sutton BJ. The allergic march from Staphylococcus aureus superantigens to immunoglobulin E. *Chem Immunol Allergy*. 2007;93:106-36.

82. Agache I, Duca L, Anghel M, Pamfil G. Antinuclear antibodies in asthma patients- a special asthma phenotype? *Iran J Allergy Asthma Immunol*. 2009;8:49-52.

83. Lee HA, Kwon B, Hur GY, Choi SJ, Nahm DH, Park HS. Isotype and IgG subclass distribution of autoantibody response to alpha-enolase protein in adult patients with severe asthma. *Yonsei Med J*. 2008;49:923-30.

84. Nahm DH, Lee KH, Shin JY, Ye YM, Kang Y, Park HS. Identification of alpha-enolase as an autoantigen associated with severe asthma. *J Allergy Clin Immunol*. 2006;118:376-81.

85. Zehn D, Bevan MJ, Fink PJ. Cutting edge: TCR revision affects predominantly Foxp3 cells and skews them toward the Th17 lineage. *J Immunol*. 2007;179:5653-7.

86. Ou LS, Goleva E, Hall C, Leung DY. T regulatory cells in atopic dermatitis and subversion of their activity by superantigens. *J Allergy Clin Immunol*. 2004;113:756-63.

87. Cardona ID, Goleva E, Ou LS, Leung DY. Staphylococcal enterotoxin B inhibits regulatory T cells by inducing glucocorticoid-induced TNF receptor-related protein ligand on monocytes. *J Allergy Clin Immunol*. 2006;117:688-95.

88. Guiducci C, Gong M, Xu Z, Gill M, Chaussabel D, Meeker T, et al. TLR recognition of self nucleic acids hampers glucocorticoid activity in lupus. *Nature*. 2010;465:937-41.

89. Okamoto K, Tanaka H, Ogawa H, Makino Y, Eguchi H, Hayashi S, et al. Redox-dependent regulation of nuclear import of the glucocorticoid receptor. *J Biol Chem.* 1999;274:10363-71.

90. Rahman I, Adcock IM. Oxidative stress and redox regulation of lung inflammation in COPD. *Eur Respir J.* 2006;28:219-42.

91. Usmani OS, Ito K, Maneechotesuwan K, Ito M, Johnson M, Barnes PJ, et al. Glucocorticoid receptor nuclear translocation in airway cells after inhaled combination therapy. *Am J Respir Crit Care Med.* 2005;172:704-12.

92. Adcock IM, Ford PA, Bhavsar P, Ahmad T, Chung KF. Steroid resistance in asthma: mechanisms and treatment options. *Curr Allergy Asthma Rep.* 2008;8:171-8.

93. Roth M, Black JL. Transcription factors in asthma: are transcription factors a new target for asthma therapy? *Curr Drug Targets.* 2006;7:589-95.

94. Loke TK, Mallett KH, Ratoff J, O'Connor BJ, Ying S, Meng Q, et al. Systemic glucocorticoid reduces bronchial mucosal activation of activator protein 1 components in glucocorticoid-sensitive but not glucocorticoid-resistant asthmatic patients. *J Allergy Clin Immunol.* 2006;118:368-75.

95. Barnes PJ, Dweik RA, Gelb AF, Gibson PG, George SC, Grasemann H, et al. Exhaled nitric oxide in pulmonary diseases: a comprehensive review. *Chest.* 2010;138:682-92.

96. Galigniana MD, Piwien-Pilipuk G, Assreuy J. Inhibition of glucocorticoid receptor binding by nitric oxide. *Mol Pharmacol.* 1999;55:317-23.

97. Paul-Clark MJ, Roviezzo F, Flower RJ, Cirino G, Soldato PD, Adcock IM, et al. Glucocorticoid receptor nitration leads to enhanced anti-inflammatory effects of novel steroid ligands. *J Immunol.* 2003;171:3245-52.

98. Nott A, Watson PM, Robinson JD, Crepaldi L, Riccio A. S-Nitrosylation of histone deacetylase 2 induces chromatin remodelling in neurons. *Nature.* 2008;455:411-5.

99. Osoata GO, Yamamura S, Ito M, Vuppusetty C, Adcock IM, Barnes PJ, et al. Nitration of distinct tyrosine residues causes inactivation of histone deacetylase 2. *Biochem Biophys Res Commun.* 2009;384:366-71

100. Hew M, Bhavsar P, Torrego A, Meah S, Khorasani N, Barnes PJ, et al. Relative corticosteroid insensitivity of peripheral blood mononuclear cells in severe asthma. *Am J Respir Crit Care Med.* 2006;174:134-41.

101. Bergeron C, Fukakusa M, Olivenstein R, Lemiere C, Shannon J, Ernst P, et al. Increased glucocorticoid receptor-beta expression, but not decreased histone deacetylase 2, in severe asthma. *J Allergy Clin Immunol.* 2006;117:703-5.

102. Barnes PJ. Targeting the epigenome in the treatment of asthma and chronic obstructive pulmonary disease. *Proc Am Thorac Soc.* 2009;6:693-6.

103. Bartling TR, Drumm ML. Loss of CFTR results in reduction of histone deacetylase 2 in airway epithelial cells. *Am J Physiol Lung Cell Mol Physiol.* 2009;297:L35-43.

104. Adcock IM, Ford P, Ito K, Barnes PJ. Epigenetics and airways disease. *Respir Res.* 2006;7:21.

105. Ford PA, Durham AL, Russell RE, Gordon F, Adcock IM, Barnes PJ. Treatment effects of low-dose theophylline combined with an inhaled corticosteroid in COPD. *Chest.* 2010;137:1338-44.

106. Marwick JA, Caramori G, Stevenson CS, Casolari P, Jazrawi E, Barnes PJ, et al. Inhibition of PI3Kdelta restores glucocorticoid function in smoking-induced airway inflammation in mice. *Am J Respir Crit Care Med.* 2009;179:542-8.

107. To Y, Ito K, Kizawa Y, Failla M, Ito M, Kusama T, et al. Targeting phosphoinositide-3-kinase-delta with theophylline reverses corticosteroid insensitivity in chronic obstructive pulmonary disease. *Am J Respir Crit Care Med.* 2010;182:897-904.

108. Marks PA. Discovery and development of SAHA as an anticancer agent. *Oncogene*. 2007;26:1351-6.

109. Aoyagi S, Archer TK. Modulating molecular chaperone Hsp90 functions through reversible acetylation. *Trends Cell Biol*. 2005;15:565-7.

110. Kovacs JJ, Murphy PJ, Gaillard S, Zhao X, Wu JT, Nicchitta CV, et al. HDAC6 regulates Hsp90 acetylation and chaperone-dependent activation of glucocorticoid receptor. *Mol Cell*. 2005;18:601-7.

111. Jee YK, Gilmour J, Kelly A, Bowen H, Richards D, Soh C, et al. Repression of interleukin-5 transcription by the glucocorticoid receptor targets GATA3 signaling and involves histone deacetylase recruitment. *J Biol Chem*. 2005;280:23243-50.

112. Hong W, Baniahmad A, Li J, Chang C, Gao W, Liu Y. Bag-1M inhibits the transactivation of the glucocorticoid receptor via recruitment of corepressors. *FEBS Lett*. 2009;583:2451-6.

113. Amat R, Solanes G, Giralt M, Villarroya F. SIRT1 is involved in glucocorticoid-mediated control of uncoupling protein-3 gene transcription. *J Biol Chem*. 2007;282:34066-76.

114. Islam KN, Mendelson CR. Glucocorticoid/glucocorticoid receptor inhibition of surfactant protein-A (SP-A) gene expression in lung type II cells is mediated by repressive changes in histone modification at the SP-A promoter. *Mol Endocrinol*. 2008;22:585-96.

115. Lander ES. Initial impact of the sequencing of the human genome. *Nature*. 2011;470:187-97.

116. Obeidat M, Hall IP. Genetics of complex respiratory diseases: implications for pathophysiology and pharmacology studies. *Br J Pharmacol*. 2011;163:96-105.

117. Swarr DT, Hakonarson H. Unraveling the complex genetic underpinnings of asthma and allergic disorders. *Curr Opin Allergy Clin Immunol*. 2010;10:434-42.

118. Kabesch M. Next generation genetics in allergy. *Curr Opin Allergy Clin Immunol*. 2010;10:407.

119. Bel EH. Clinical phenotypes of asthma. *Curr Opin Pulm Med*. 2004;10:44-50.

120. Fitzpatrick AM, Teague WG, Meyers DA, Peters SP, Li X, Li H, et al. Heterogeneity of severe asthma in childhood: confirmation by cluster analysis of children in the National Institutes of Health/National Heart, Lung, and Blood Institute Severe Asthma Research Program. *J Allergy Clin Immunol*. 2011;127:382-9.e1-13.

121. Moffatt MF, Kabesch M, Liang L, Dixon AL, Strachan D, Heath S, et al. Genetic variants regulating ORMDL3 expression contribute to the risk of childhood asthma. *Nature*. 2007;448:470-3.

122. Moffatt MF, Gut IG, Demenais F, Strachan DP, Bouzigon E, Heath S, et al. A large-scale, consortium-based genomewide association study of asthma. *N Engl J Med*. 2010;363:1211-21.

123. Cantero-Recasens G, Fandos C, Rubio-Moscardo F, Valverde MA, Vicente R. The asthma-associated ORMDL3 gene product regulates endoplasmic reticulum-mediated calcium signaling and cellular stress. *Hum Mol Genet*. 2010;19:111-21.

124. Creed TJ, Probert CS, Norman MN, Moorghen M, Shepherd NA, Hearing SD, et al. Basiliximab for the treatment of steroid-resistant ulcerative colitis: further experience in moderate and severe disease. *Aliment Pharmacol Ther*. 2006;23:1435-42.

125. Hurley DM, Accili D, Stratakis CA, Karl M, Vamvakopoulos N, Rorer E, et al. Point mutation causing a single amino acid substitution in the hormone binding domain of the glucocorticoid receptor in familial glucocorticoid resistance. *J Clin Invest*. 1991;87:680-6.

126. Vingerhoeds AC, Thijssen JH, Schwarz F. Spontaneous hypercortisolism without Cushing's syndrome. *J Clin Endocrinol Metab*. 1976;43:1128-33.

127. Charmandari E, Kino T, Ichijo T, Chrousos GP. Generalized glucocorticoid resistance: clinical aspects, molecular mechanisms, and implications of a rare genetic disorder. *J Clin Endocrinol Metab.* 2008;93:1563-72.

128. Huizenga NA, Koper JW, De Lange P, Pols HA, Stolk RP, Burger H, et al. A polymorphism in the glucocorticoid receptor gene may be associated with and increased sensitivity to glucocorticoids in vivo. *J Clin Endocrinol Metab.* 1998;83:144-51.

129. Kino T, Stauber RH, Resau JH, Pavlakis GN, Chrousos GP. Pathologic human GR mutant has a transdominant negative effect on the wild-type GR by inhibiting its translocation into the nucleus: importance of the ligand-binding domain for intracellular GR trafficking. *J Clin Endocrinol Metab.* 2001;86:5600-8.

130. Moore WC, Bleecker ER, Curran-Everett D, Erzurum SC, Ameredes BT, Bacharier L, et al. Characterization of the severe asthma phenotype by the National Heart, Lung, and Blood Institute's Severe Asthma Research Program. *J Allergy Clin Immunol.* 2007; 119:405-13.

131. Haldar P, Brightling CE, Hargadon B, Gupta S, Monteiro W, Sousa A, et al. Mepolizumab and exacerbations of refractory eosinophilic asthma. *N Engl J Med.* 2009;360:973-84.

132. Nair P, Pizzichini MM, Kjarsgaard M, Inman MD, Efthimiadis A, Pizzichini E, et al. Mepolizumab for prednisone-dependent asthma with sputum eosinophilia. *N Engl J Med.* 2009;360:985-93.

133. Wenzel S, Wilbraham D, Fuller R, Getz EB, Longphre M. Effect of an interleukin-4 variant on late phase asthmatic response to allergen challenge in asthmatic patients: results of two phase 2a studies. *Lancet.* 2007;370:1422-31.

134. Wenzel SE, Barnes PJ, Bleecker ER, Bousquet J, Busse W, Dahlén SE, et al. A randomized, double-blind, placebo-controlled study of tumor necrosis factor-alpha blockade in severe persistent asthma. *Am J Respir Crit Care Med.* 2009;179:549-58.

135. Goleva E, Hauk PJ, Hall CF, Liu AH, Riches DW, Martin RJ, et al. Corticosteroid-resistant asthma is associated with classical antimicrobial activation of airway macrophages. *J Allergy Clin Immunol.* 2008;122:550-9.e3.

136. Bellettato C, Adcock IM, Ito K, Caramori G, Casolari P, Ciaccia A, et al. Rhinovirus infection reduces glucocorticoid receptor nuclear translocation in airway epithelial cells. *Eur Respir J.* 2003;22:565S.

137. Garn H, Mittermann I, Valenta R, Renz H. Autosensitization as a pathomechanism in asthma. *Ann N Y Acad Sci.* 2007;1107:417-25.

Monitoring and Natural History of Refractory Asthma

10

Christopher Brightling

INTRODUCTION

Asthma affects an estimated 300 million people worldwide, and the burden is likely to rise substantially in the next few decades.[1] Approximately 5–10% of these asthmatics have severe asthma, whereby sufferers have persistent symptoms and exacerbations inspite of high-dose standard therapy.[1,2] Patients with inadequately controlled severe persistent asthma are at a particularly high risk of exacerbations, hospitalization and death, and often have severely impaired quality of life. Although this group represents a relatively small proportion of the asthma population, they consume two-thirds of the healthcare costs attributed to asthma. This disproportionate use of healthcare resources reflects a considerable unmet need to the individual patients, and to healthcare providers.

Asthma is a complex disease characterized by typical symptoms of breathlessness, wheeze, and cough together with episodes of marked worsening of symptoms known as exacerbations. These symptoms occur on a background of disordered airway physiology characterized by variable airflow limitation, airway hyper-responsiveness (AHR), and in more severe disease persistent airflow obstruction. In spite of our increasing understanding of the immunopathogenesis of asthma, there has been a paucity of novel therapies for asthma over the last 20 years. Indeed, the mainstay of therapy for asthma remains inhaled corticosteroids (ICS) and long-acting bronchodilators.[2] These therapies reduce but do not eliminate the impact of day-to-day symptoms and the frequency of exacerbations. Importantly, decline in lung function and development of airflow obstruction remain refractory to current therapy.

There is an increasing recognition that asthma encompasses several underlying pathological processes, which develop as a consequence of a variety of gene-environment interactions that give rise to a clinical phenotype. Novel developments in the measurement of airway inflammation, lung physiology and imaging, coupled with emerging data utilizing 'omic' technology and biostatistical modeling[3,4] mean that we are now positioned to inform our understanding of the complexity of airway disease. The concept that 'one size does not fit all' is also exemplified by the heterogeneity in treatment response. This variability of response to therapies will be further magnified in the context of highly specific treatments. This heterogeneity is further compounded by the increasing cost of these novel therapies, which are likely to be restricted to severe disease where the potential health economic benefit is greatest. There is therefore a pressing need to be able to unravel the complexity of asthma in order to understand structure-function relationships, disease etiology, and progression.

This chapter will summarize our current understanding of the natural history of severe asthma, outline concepts in monitoring disease, define its current clinical utility, and speculate on the future opportunities in predicting natural history and treatment response towards the goal of personalized healthcare.

NATURAL HISTORY OF ASTHMA

Asthma in Children

Asthma commonly begins in infants with an incidence of 3% of definite or probable asthma in the first year of life,[5] which falls to about 0.1% after the age of 15 years. Perhaps, the most informative study on the natural history of asthma is the Melbourne 1957 birth-cohort.[6] Children were enrolled at the age of 7 years and were categorized into 5 groups: (i) control, never wheezed; (ii) mild wheezy bronchitis, fewer than 5 episodes; (iii) wheezy bronchitis, 5 or more episodes; (iv) asthma, not associated with infection; and (v) severe asthma, onset before the age of 3 years and persistent symptoms. These subjects were reviewed regularly until aged 42. By age 42 years, some of the subjects in each group were free of asthma, and some had frequent or persistent asthma. Interestingly, the more severe the asthma at the age of 7 years, the more likely it was to persist to age 42 years (Table 10-1). Reduced lung function at the age of 7 years was associated with continuing symptoms in adult life, and the lung function continued to be reduced but did not appear to decline more rapidly than the control or mild groups with normal forced expiratory volume in 1 second (FEV_1) or progress to airflow obstruction. Presence of hay fever, eczema, or positive skin test results increased the risk of more severe asthma in adult life.

Table 10-1	Study of Childhood Asthma: Outcome at the Age of 42 Years of the 4 Groups Classified by Severity at the Age of 7 Years (% of group)[6]			
Control level	Mild wheezy bronchitis	Wheezy bronchitis	Asthma	Severe asthma
No recent asthma	68	58	32	10
Infrequent asthma	18	15	18	13
Frequent asthma	17	17	26	27
Persistent asthma	0	10	24	50

These observations have been confirmed and extended by other cohorts, including Tucson,[7] Dunedin,[8] Denver,[9] London,[10] and the Isle of Wight.[11] Together these studies suggest that the predictors of persistent and severe childhood asthma are more severe and include frequent wheezing episodes during preschool age, onset during school age, family history of asthma and allergy, although no clear genetic determinant of progression has been identified, elevated serum IgE, early evidence of sensitization, early AHR, frequent respiratory tract infections, and lack of contact with older children.

Asthma in Adults

Asthma may persist from childhood or initiates in adult life. The primary variable for persistence and severity of asthma identified in longitudinal studies is the severity in childhood. Francis Rackemann, who introduced the concept of intrinsic asthma in the 1920s, reported in 1958 a follow-up study of his patients with adult-onset non-allergic asthma and only about 20% had a remission.[12] The Tucson study showed that remissions were uncommon after the second decade, and were especially uncommon in subjects 30–60 years old. Relapses of asthma that began at any age were common and increased until age 70 years.[13] Lung function of some, but no means all, adult patients with asthma declines over the years.[14-16] One study evaluating the decline of FEV_1 reported that although aerosol glucocorticoid treatment improved FEV_1, it did not prevent continued deterioration. Patients in the Third National Health and Nutrition Examination Survey of 1063 adults, 20 years of age or older, with lifelong history of asthma had deterioration of lung function; but this included subjects with airway obstruction and restriction.[17] There are many reasons for this deterioration of lung function including airway remodeling from persistent inflammation or environmental exposure, such as smoking. Allergic bronchopulmonary aspergillosis frequently causes permanent loss of lung function, because of bronchiectasis and segmental fibrosis.[18] Bronchiectasis can also coexist with asthma in the absence of sensitization to *Aspergillus fumigatus*,[19] and *Aspergillus fumigatus* sensitization is associated with poor lung function even in the absence of bronchiectasis.[20]

MONITORING SEVERE ASTHMA CONTROL AND RISK

The ultimate aim of asthma management is cure, but to date, this has eluded asthma specialists. Therefore, the current aim of asthma management is to achieve disease control in terms of symptoms and functional limitations, minimize future risk of exacerbations, and disease progression whilst avoiding unnecessary therapies and their potential side effects.[1,2,21,22] Monitoring severe asthma thus requires measures of symptom control, health status, exacerbations, disease progression, and responsiveness to therapy. Measurements of the underlying biological processes, including inflammation, remodeling, and environment exposure can define the disease within individuals and are beginning to help direct therapies and to stratify future risk.

Table 10-2	Level of Asthma Control in Patients ≥5 Years of Age. Any of the Components Places the Patient in the Category		
Control level	*Well controlled***	*Partially controlled***	*Poorly controlled***
Daytime symptoms in the past 2–4 weeks	≤2 days/week but not more than once a day	>2 days/week or more than once a day but ≤2 days/week	Throughout the day
Limitations of activities in the past 2–4 weeks	None	Some limitation	Extremely limited
Nocturnal symptoms/awakenings in the past 2–4 weeks	None	≤2 nights/week	>2 nights/week
Need for short-acting inhaled β_2-agonists in the past 2–4 weeks	≤2 days/week	>2 days/week	Several times a day
Lung function FEV_1 or PEFR* FEV_1/FVC (<11 years of age)	≥80% predicted or personal best ≥80%	60–79% predicted or personal best 75–80%	<60% predicted or personal best <75%
Exacerbation(s) (requiring oral or systemic corticosteroids)***	0–1/year	2/year	Frequent (>2/year)
	Consider severity and interval since last exacerbation		

*FEV_1 or PEF may be ≥80% predicted in patients with severe persistent asthma
**For well-controlled asthma, all components should be present; for partially or poorly controlled asthma, any of the components places the patient in the category
***At present, there are inadequate data to correspond frequencies of exacerbations with different levels of asthma control of severity.
FEV_1, forced expiratory volume in 1 second; FVC, forced vital capacity.
Adapted from Bousquet J, Mantzouranis E, Cruz A, Aït-Khaled N, Baena-Cagnani CE, Bleecker ER, et al. Uniform definition of asthma severity, control, and exacerbations: document presented for the World Health Organization consultation. *J Allergy Clin Immunol.* 2010;126:926-38.

Control

The level of asthma control incorporates current clinical control and exacerbations (Table 10-2). Current clinical control or extent of impairment is the frequency and intensity of symptoms and functional limitations that a patient experiences or has recently experienced as a consequence of asthma. It includes measures of day and night symptoms, use of reliever therapy, activity limitations, and lung function. The time period for which current clinical control should be assessed is proposed to be the previous 2–4 weeks for adults and at least 4 weeks for children. The number of asthma exacerbations requiring oral systemic corticosteroids (high-dose for over 3 days) in the previous year should also be considered in evaluating overall asthma control.[23]

Until recently, strong emphasis has been placed on lung function measures, such as peak expiratory flow (PEF) and FEV$_1$, before and after a bronchodilator, as a measure of asthma control or asthma severity. There is an inconsistent relationship between lung function measures and symptoms or exacerbation frequency as patient-centered outcome measures.[24] Therefore, it is important for a comprehensive assessment to capture multiple asthma endpoints, including lung function.

Questionnaires for assessing asthma control have been developed. These tools score asthma indices as continuous variables and thus provide numerical values to distinguish different levels of control [(e.g., Asthma Control Test (ACT),[25] Childhood Asthma Control Test, Asthma Control Questionnaire (ACQ)[26]].

Risk

The concept of asthma risk[1] captures the likelihood of asthma exacerbations, development of chronic morbidity including progressive loss of pulmonary function over time, or the risk of adverse reactions from asthma medication.[27]

Exacerbations are episodes of progressive increase in shortness of breath, cough, wheezing, and chest tightness, or a combination of these symptoms. The exacerbation frequency is a measure of control, as described above, and future exacerbations represent a risk. The exacerbation frequency is a good predictor of this future risk. Exacerbations are characterized by decreases in expiratory airflow (PEF or FEV$_1$). However, PEF variability does not usually increase during an exacerbation although may do so leading up to or during the recovery from an exacerbation.[28] The severity of exacerbations ranges from mild to life threatening and can be evaluated based on both symptoms and lung function. Exacerbations should be considered separately from current clinical control when evaluating overall asthma control because exacerbations may occur in a patient even if the patient has adequate day-to-day control of symptoms and minimal activity limitations. Such exacerbations may or may not be prevented by escalating maintenance therapy.

Response to therapy in terms of achieving control or reducing risk is variable and is likely to be dependent upon the underlying biology that determines the phenotype of individual patients. For example, response to anti-inflammatory therapy may be predictable by measuring the relevant biological pathway in patients.

MONITORING INFLAMMATION IN SEVERE ASTHMA

Several tools are available to measure airway inflammation noninvasively including exhaled breath analysis, breath condensate, and sputum analysis as well as invasive measures such as bronchoscopic sampling. To date, sputum differential cell counts (Figure 10-1) and fractional exhaled nitric oxide (FeNO) are the most widely explored.[29]

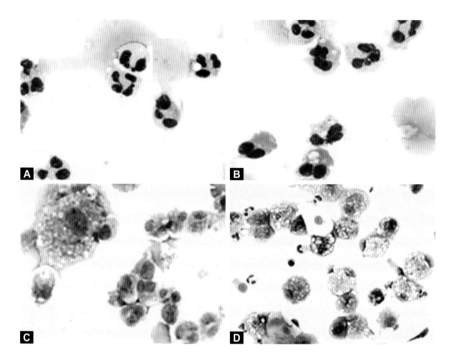

Figure 10-1 Sputum cytospins from different subjects with asthma illustrate the heterogeneity of the airway inflammation. **A,** Predominant cells are macrophages with a normal neutrophil and eosinophil count; this cytospin cannot be distinguished from a sample from a healthy control subject (paucigranulocytic asthma, original ×100). **B,** Combined neutrophilic and eosinophilic inflammation (original ×400). **C,** Neutrophilic inflammation (original ×400). **D,** Eosinophilic inflammation (original ×400). *From* Brightling CE. Clinical applications of induced sputum. *Chest.* 2006;129:1344-8; *with permission.*

Targeted Corticosteroid Therapy

Inhaled corticosteroids have been the mainstay of anti-inflammatory treatment for asthma since the 1970s, and a number of placebo-controlled trials have convincingly demonstrated a reduction in exacerbation frequency across the spectrum of severity, as recently reviewed.[30] However, there remains the possibility that this benefit may be largely confined to a subgroup of asthmatic patients, and indeed recent studies have shown that the major benefit occurs in patients with eosinophilic airway inflammation,[31] while the subgroup with predominantly neutrophilic airway inflammation respond poorly.[32] Importantly, the value of measuring airway inflammation in sputum extends beyond these relatively short-term studies on corticosteroid responsiveness. Corticosteroid reduction studies have shown that a sputum eosinophilia develops well before the onset of an exacerbation[33,34] suggesting that targeted therapy in asthma aimed at normalizing the sputum eosinophil count could lead to a reduction in asthma exacerbations.

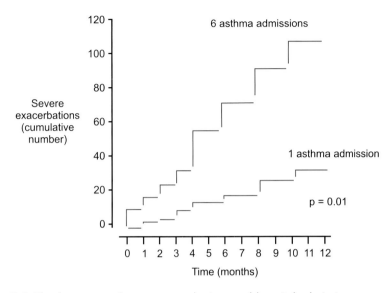

Figure 10-2 The frequency of severe exacerbations and hospital admissions over one year were reduced in severe asthmatics managed using sputum eosinophil directed therapy compared to standard guideline. *Adapted from* Green RH, Brightling CE, McKenna S, Hargadon B, Parker D, Bradding P, et al. Asthma exacerbations and sputum eosinophil counts: a randomized controlled trial. *Lancet.* 2002;360:1715-21; *with permission.*

Three randomized controlled trials have compared standard guideline-based asthma management with sputum-based management in which ICS dose was titrated according to the sputum eosinophil count.[35-37] In a randomized placebo-controlled trial, 74 subjects with asthma were assigned to either a management strategy aimed at normalizing their sputum eosinophil count or standard clinical care.[35] Patients in the sputum management group experienced significantly fewer severe asthma exacerbations than patients in the control group (35 vs. 109; p = 0.01) (Figure 10-2) and significantly fewer patients were admitted to hospital with asthma (1 vs. 6; p = 0.047). The reduction in exacerbations was achieved without an increase in the total corticosteroid dose in the sputum guidelines group as monitoring airway inflammation in the sputum guidelines group identified a group of patients with noneosinophilic asthma whose sputum eosinophil count remained within the normal range and in these subjects the dose of corticosteroids was reduced without evidence of deterioration in control. In a second study of 117 asthmatics entered into a 2-year follow-up multicenter, randomized, parallel group effectiveness study,[36] treatment directed at normalizing the sputum eosinophil count also led to a reduction in exacerbations (79 vs. 47; p = 0.04) and increased the time to first exacerbation by 213 days. This benefit was not at the expense of increased therapy in the intervention group. In this study, the inflammatory phenotype of the exacerbations were characterized and in the sputum guidelines group eosinophilic, but not noneosinophilic exacerbations were reduced. Interestingly, the noneosinophilic exacerbations were more common (56%). The reduction in exacerbations was more apparent in those with severe disease. This suggests that it is probably most appropriate to apply this technique to the management of difficult-to-treat or refractory asthma, but that its use may not be generalizable to a primary care population.

A meta-analysis concluded that sputum-based strategies were effective in reducing exacerbations in adults with asthma without a net increase in mean ICS dose.[38,39] Furthermore, Haldar et al. showed that the sputum-based strategy was of particular benefit in certain subgroups of asthmatic patients.[3] Most notably, a "discordant inflammation" group was identified in whom eosinophilic inflammation occurred in the absence of severe symptoms. Uptitration of ICS in order to control sputum eosinophilia resulted in a markedly reduced exacerbation rate. Conversely, the "discordant symptom" group were severely symptomatic despite the absence of eosinophilic airway inflammation. ICS could be reduced in this group without an increase in exacerbation rate.

The inclusion of sputum induction in the management of asthma is cost effective. Economic analysis shows that the healthcare-related savings as a consequence of the reduction in asthma exacerbations outweighs the cost of sputum induction and processing.[35] Sputum induction is relatively labor intensive and requires laboratory support, but all of the equipment is available in a routine pathology laboratory and minimal training is required. Therefore, sputum induction should be available as a routine test in specialist centers to evaluate and manage patients with severe asthma.

Management strategies based on FeNO, a surrogate marker of eosinophilic airway inflammation, have been less successful. A recent meta-analysis of six randomized controlled trials (two in adults and four in children/adolescents) concluded that a FeNO-based strategy did not result in a significantly different exacerbation rate compared to standard management.[38,39]

Targeted Novel Anti-inflammatory Therapies

Accurate disease phenotyping has assumed greater importance with the emergence of biological therapies that target very specific components of the immune response. Treatments are likely to be effective only in a subset of patients with asthma and are currently in phase I-III clinical trials. Some are moving closer to the clinic, such as those targeting the Th2 cytokines, interleukin (IL)-4, -5, and -13.

IL-5 is known to be a major player in eosinophilic airway inflammation through its actions of promoting eosinophil production, maturation, activation, and survival. An initial randomized controlled trial of mepolizumab, a monoclonal anti-IL-5 antibody, in 362 unselected patients with persistent asthma found no statistically significant clinical benefit, although there was a trend towards a reduction in exacerbation rates.[40] However, two later trials found that in patients with refractory eosinophilic asthma despite high-dose inhaled or oral corticosteroids, mepolizumab significantly reduced rates of exacerbations,[41,42] improved Asthma Quality of Life Questionnaire (AQLQ) scores,[41] and allowed oral prednisolone doses to be successfully reduced.[42]

Pitrakinra, an IL-4 variant, reduced the allergen-induced late-phase response and the need for rescue medication in asthmatic patients.[43] Recent evidence in a phase II study suggests that efficacy is greatest in those with eosinophilic inflammation. AMG-317 is a fully human monoclonal antibody to IL-4Rα that blocks both IL-4 and IL-13 pathways and was administered to mainly healthy adults and a smaller number of asthmatic adults, and earlier studies have established its bioavailability and safety. Recently a phase II, randomized, double-blind, placebo-controlled study of AMG-317 in 147 moderate-to-severe asthmatics[44] showed an improvement in the number and time to exacerbation in the treatment arm. The study failed to meet its primary endpoint of improvement in asthma control. The drug was however well tolerated and there was improvement in those patients with poor control as baseline. Whether IL-4 and IL-13 strategies need to target eosinophilic, atopic or poorly controlled patients is uncertain, but it remains likely that there are sub-populations that may respond well to these therapies and there remains a need to identify biomarkers of response.

MONITORING ENVIRONMENTAL EXPOSURE IN SEVERE ASTHMA

Anti-IgE

Omalizumab is a humanized anti-IgE monoclonal antibody. A systematic review of eight placebo-controlled trials of omalizumab in moderate or severe allergic asthma showed that omalizumab reduced exacerbation frequency and facilitated corticosteroid withdrawal.[45] The use of omalizumab is currently restricted to patients with severe uncontrolled allergic asthma with raised IgE levels and a positive skin prick test to a perennial allergen.[46] Although a recent case report suggested that benefit may not be restricted to patients with positive skin prick tests,[47] this has not been confirmed in larger-scale studies.

Antifungal Therapy

Allergic bronchopulmonary aspergillosis (ABPA) is a relatively uncommon condition in which long-term colonization of the airways with, and sensitization to, the fungus *Aspergillus fumigatus* results in airway inflammation and bronchiectasis, usually in association with asthma. Previous studies have shown that treatment with itraconazole is beneficial in this group of patients.[48-51] More recently, it has been hypothesized that ABPA may form just one end of a spectrum of airway disease associated with fungal sensitization, and that severe asthma with fungal sensitization (SAFS) may be a distinct asthma phenotype with therapeutic implications.[51] *Aspergillus fumigatus* IgE sensitization and airway colonization are associated with reduced FEV_1 in patients with asthma.[20] A randomized controlled trial of itraconazole in 58 patients with SAFS, but not ABPA showed a significant improvement in the AQLQ scores in the treatment arm, as well as in the rhinitis scores and morning peak flow readings.[52]

Macrolide Antibiotics

Macrolides are known to possess anti-inflammatory properties over and above their antimicrobial activity,[53] and they are of proven benefit in diffuse panbronchiolitis.[54] Clinical trials of macrolides in asthmatics have yielded conflicting results with no definite overall benefit.[55] However, there is evidence that macrolides may specifically target neutrophilic airway inflammation. A recent study of 45 patients with refractory asthma found that 8 weeks of treatment with clarithromycin (500 mg twice daily) resulted in significantly reduced levels of sputum IL-8, reduced airway neutrophil numbers, and improved quality of life scores compared to placebo.[56] These differences were more marked in the subgroup of patients with noneosinophilic asthma, suggesting that macrolides may be employed as a targeted therapy in this group.

MONITORING DISEASE PROGRESSION AND REMODELING IN SEVERE ASTHMA

Disease progression is typically measured by FEV_1 decline, but encompasses several processes affecting small and large airway wall and caliber and mechanics. This is largely due to airway remodeling. Airway remodeling is associated with disease severity, air flow limitation, airway hyper-responsiveness,[57] and eosinophilic inflammation.[58] Airway remodeling consists of an increase in smooth muscle mass due to hyperplastic and hypertrophic changes, mucous gland hyperplasia, thickening of reticular basement membrane, dysregulated extracellular matrix deposition, and increased vasculature[59] in both the large and the small airways.[60]

The identification of remodeling patterns in various phenotypes of severe asthma and the ability to relate airway structure to important clinical outcomes, airway physiology, and inflammation would help close a crucial gap in our understanding of severe asthma phenotypes, and could help target treatment more effectively. Recent advances in imaging technology now permit detailed assessment of large and small airway architecture, evaluation of lung parenchyma, as well as, the ability to perform functional and physiological evaluations[61-63] (Figures 10-3 and 10-4). Furthermore,

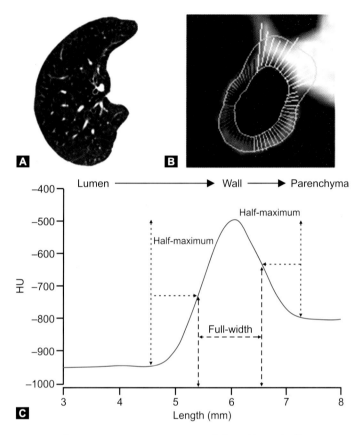

Figure 10-3 Airway dimension estimation using full-width at half maximum principle. **A,** A representative computed tomography image is shown. **B,** A magnified view of an airway is shown. Rays can be seen between the inner and outer boundary of the airway wall. Some rays extend into the pulmonary artery because the artery has similar X-ray attenuation values as the airway wall. Those rays are manually eliminated and the airway dimension calculated using the remaining rays. **C,** A representative X-ray attenuation profile for a ray that passes from airway lumen to the lung parenchyma through the airway wall is shown. The inner and outer airway wall boundary is estimated based on points at which X-ray attenuation value is half way to the local maximum and half way to the local minimum, respectively. *From* Siddiqui S, Gupta S, Cruse G, Haldar P, Entwisle J, Mcdonald S, et al. Airway wall geometry in asthma and nonasthmatic eosinophilic bronchitis. *Allergy.* 2009;64:951-8; *with permission.*

novel techniques are emerging that will allow us to observe inflammation profiles and molecular pathways in severe asthma to further enhance our understanding of the structure-function relationship. Indeed, recent findings in severe asthma have related airway remodeling identified by CT to eosinophilic and neutrophilic inflammation over time with poor lung function[63] (Figure 10-5). Airway wall

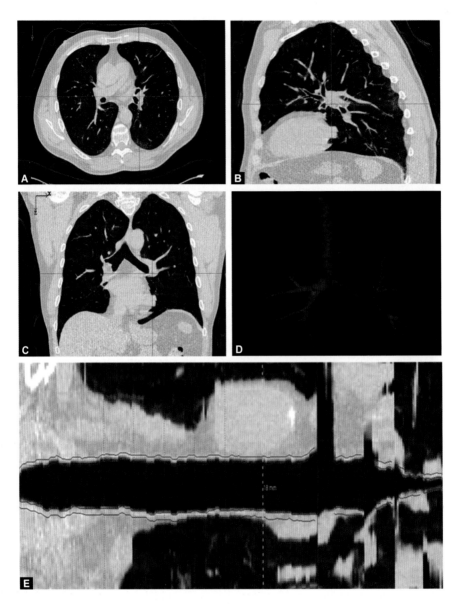

Figure 10-4 A screen shot of the Pulmonary Workstation 2.0 software (VIDA Diagnostics). This software uses the maximum-likelihood method to perform three-dimensional analysis of the airway tree on volumetric CT scan. **A–C,** The longitudinal section of the reformatted airway is shown. **D,** The three-dimensional reconstruction of the airway tree. **E,** Measurements of the airway dimensions are automatically calculated for each segment of the airway path (between airway branch points) as indicated by the red lines at the level of the inferior lobar bronchus.

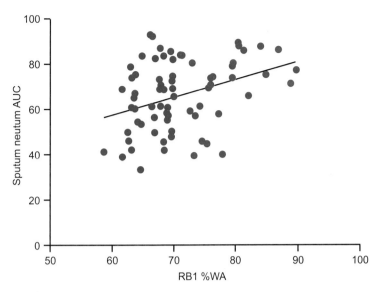

Figure 10-5 Correlation between right upper lobe apical segmental bronchus (RB1) percentage wall area (%WA) and sputum neutrophil area under the curve (AUC %) in patients with severe asthma (r = 0.36, p < 0.005). *From* Gupta S, Siddiqui S, Haldar P, Entwisle JJ, Mawby D, Wardlaw AJ, et al. Quantitative analysis of high-resolution computed tomography scans in severe asthma subphenotypes. *Thorax.* 2010;65:775-81; *with permission.*

thickening assessed by CT also improved following mepolizumab therapy,[41] suggesting that modulating eosinophilic inflammation may impact upon airway remodeling and importantly that imaging may be an important tool to stratify patients and to assess clinical outcomes.

PREDICTING THE FUTURE: DISEASE PROGRESSION AND RESPONSE TO THERAPY

Statistical Modeling of Airway Disease: Phenotyping the Heterogeneity

Early observational studies have identified clinical and pathological features associated with persistent airflow obstruction and exacerbation frequency using multiple regression.[64,65] The integration of data derived from noninvasive markers of airway inflammation have provided new inflammatory phenotypes of eosinophilic and noneosinophilic asthma[29] and further statistical modeling using factor and cluster analysis has provided further insight into the complexity of asthma phenotypes.[3]

The integration of data now available from multiple scales potentially, including the genome and transcriptome can be used to develop statistical models of future risk to develop frequent exacerbations, lung function decline, or likelihood to respond to therapy. Using a variety of data reduction methods, panels of biomarkers can and will be identified as 'fingerprints' of specific airway disease subphenotypes. To date these statistical approaches have been largely restricted to cross-sectional observations and have used tools, such as cluster analysis, which lack mathematical inference. Hence, the generalizability of these findings beyond the cohorts studied or phenotypic stability within these cohorts is unknown. Therefore, these statistical approaches remain limited in their ability to predict response to therapies and disease progression.

Patient-specific Multiscale Computational Models

Patient-specific multiscale computational models like statistical models embrace the complexity of airways disease, but also have the potential to provide insights into the interactions across multiple scales and time. Models of the respiratory system in health have been established. A smaller number of airway disease-specific models exist at the tissue-organ level of large and small airway disease[66,67] and at the molecular-cellular level for airway smooth muscle contraction.[66,68] The challenge is therefore to extend and integrate these existing models.

Thus far computational models have not realized their clinical potential. Current models have not been extensively validated in large cohorts of well-characterized patients. Therefore, their ability to predict future outcomes has not been fully defined. Furthermore, models of airway disease have not been integrated across multiple scales.

CONCLUSION

Severe asthma is a heterogeneous condition and its natural history is poorly understood. It is likely that within an individual numerous biological processes are acting in concert to impact upon and inform the clinical expression of disease. Monitoring of these domains is beginning to influence clinical outcomes. Further understanding of these complex interactions is likely to assist in the development of predictive models of disease progression and response to therapy.

REFERENCES

1. Bousquet J, Mantzouranis E, Cruz A, Aït-Khaled N, Baena-Cagnani CE, Bleecker ER, et al. Uniform definition of asthma severity, control, and exacerbations: document presented for the World Health Organisation consultation on Severe Asthma. *J Allergy Clin Immunol.* 2010;126:926-38.
2. British Thoracic Society Scottish Intercollegiate Guidelines Network. British Guideline on the Management of Asthma. *Thorax.* 2008;63:iv1-121.
3. Haldar P, Pavord ID, Shaw DE, Berry MA, Thomas M, Brightling CE, et al. Cluster analysis and clinical asthma phenotypes. *Am J Respir Crit Care Med.* 2008;178:218-24.
4. Moore WC, Meyers DA, Wenzel SE, Teague WG, Li H, Li X, et al. Identification of asthma phenotypes using cluster analysis in the Severe Asthma Research Program. *Am J Respir Crit Care Med.* 2010;181:315-23.

5. Yunginger JW, Reed CE, O'Connell EJ, Melton LJ 3rd, O'Fallon WM, Silverstein MD. A community-based study of the epidemiology of asthma. Incidence rates, 1964-1983. *Am Rev Respir Dis.* 1992;146:888-94.

6. Phelan PD, Robertson CF, Olinsky A. The Melbourne Asthma Study: 1964-1999. *J Allergy Clin Immunol.* 2002;109:189-94.

7. Taussig LM, Wright AL, Holberg CJ, Halonen M, Morgan WJ, Martinez FD. Tucson Children's Respiratory Study: 1980 to present. *J Allergy Clin Immunol.* 2003;111:661-75.

8. Jones DT, Sears MR, Holdaway MD, Hewitt CJ, Flannery EM, Herbison GP, et al. Childhood asthma in NewZealand. *Br J Dis Chest.* 1987;81:332-40.

9. Klinnert MD, Nelson HS, Price MR, Adinoff AD, Leung DY, Mrazek DA. Onset and persistence of childhood asthma: predictors from infancy. *Pediatrics.* 2001;108:E69.

10. Blair H. Natural history of childhood asthma: 20-year follow-up. *Arch Dis Child.* 1977;52: 613-9.

11. Kurukulaaratchy RJ, Matthews S, Arshad SH, Kurukulaaratchy RJ, Matthews S, Arshad SH. Defining childhood atopic phenotypes to investigate the association of atopic sensitization with allergic disease. *Allergy.* 2005;60:1280-6.

12. Rackemann FM, Edwards MC. Is intrinsic asthma a reversible disease? A follow-up study. *J Allergy.* 1958;29:528-34.

13. Bronnimann S, Burrows B. A prospective study of the natural history of asthma. Remission and relapse rates. *Chest.* 1986;90:480-4.

14. Ulrik CS. Outcome of asthma: longitudinal changes in lung function. *Eur Respir J.* 1999;13:904-18.

15. McFadden ER Jr. Natural history of chronic asthma and its long-term effects on pulmonary function. *J Allergy Clin Immunol.* 2000;105:S535-9.

16. Lange P, Parner J, Vestbo J, Schnohr P, Jensen G. A 15-year follow-up study of ventilator function in adults with asthma. *N Engl J Med.* 1998;339:1194-200.

17. Savage-Brown A, Mannino DM, Redd SC. Lung disease and asthma severity in adults with asthma: data from the Third National Health and Nutrition Examination. *J Asthma.* 2005;42:519-23.

18. Greenberger PA. Allergic bronchopulmonary aspergillosis. *J Allergy Clin Immunol.* 2002; 110:685-92.

19. Gupta S, Siddiqui S, Haldar P, Raj JV, Entwisle JJ, Wardlaw AJ, et al. Qualitative Analysis of High-Resolution CT Scans in Severe Asthma. *Chest.* 2009;136:1521-8.

20. Fairs A, Agbetile J, Hargadon B, Bourne M, Monteiro WR, Brightling CE, et al. IgE sensitization to Aspergillus fumigatus is associated with reduced lung function in asthma. *Am J Respir Crit Care Med.* 2010;182:1362-8.

21. National Asthma Education and Prevention Program. Expert Panel Report 3 (EPR3): Guidelines for the Diagnosis and Management of Asthma. Available from URL: http://www.nhlbi.nih.gov/guidelines/asthma/asthgdln.htm.

22. Global Initiative for Asthma Available from URL:www.GINA.org.

23. Taylor DR, Bateman ED, Boulet LP, Boushey HA, Busse WW, Casale TB, et al. A new perspective on concepts of asthma severity and control. *Eur Respir J.* 2008;32:545-54.

24. Moore WC, Bleecker ER, Curran-Everett D, Erzurum SC, Ameredes BT, Bacharier L, et al. Characterization of the severe asthma phenotype by the National Heart, Lung, and Blood Institute's Severe Asthma Research Program. *J Allergy Clin Immunol.* 2007;119:405-13.

25. Nathan RA, Sorkness CA, Kosinski M, Schatz M, Li JT, Marcus P, et al. Development of the asthma control test: a survey for assessing asthma control. *J Allergy Clin Immunol.* 2004;113:59-65.

26. Juniper EF, O'Byrne PM, Guyatt GH, Ferrie PJ, King DR. Development and validation of a questionnaire to measure asthma control. *Eur Respir J.* 1999;14:902-7.

27. Sullivan SD, Wenzel SE, Bresnahan BW, Zheng B, Lee JH, Pritchard M, et al. Association of control and risk of severe asthma-related events in severe or difficult-to-treat asthma patients. *Allergy.* 2007;62:655-60.

28. Reddel H, Ware S, Marks G, Salome C, Jenkins C, Woolcock A. Differences between asthma exacerbations and poor asthma control. *Lancet.* 1999;353:364-9.

29. Brightling CE. Clinical applications of induced sputum. *Chest.* 2006;129:1344-8.

30. Desai D, Siddiqui S, Brightling C. Can inhaled corticosteroids prevent asthma exacerbations? *Curr Opin Pulm Med.* 2011;17:16-22.

31. Green RH, Brightling CE, Woltmann G, Parker D, Wardlaw AJ, Pavord ID. Analysis of induced sputum in adults with asthma: identification of subgroup with isolated sputum neutrophilia and poor response to inhaled corticosteroids. *Thorax.* 2002;57:875-9.

32. Berry M, Morgan A, Shaw DE, Parker D, Green R, Brightling C, et al. Pathological features and inhaled corticosteroid response of eosinophilic and non-eosinophilic asthma. *Thorax.* 2007;62:1043-9.

33. Pizzichini MM, Pizzichini E, Clelland L, Efthimiadis A, Pavord I, Dolovich J, et al. Prednisone-dependent asthma: inflammatory indices in induced sputum. *Eur Respir J.* 1999;13:15-21.

34. Jatakanon A, Lim S, Barnes PJ. Changes in sputum eosinophils predict loss of asthma control. *Am J Respir Crit Care Med.* 2000;161:64-72.

35. Green RH, Brightling CE, McKenna S, Hargadon B, Parker D, Bradding P, et al. Asthma exacerbations and sputum eosinophil counts: a randomized controlled trial. *Lancet.* 2002;360:1715-21.

36. Chlumský J, Striz I, Terl M, Vondracek J. Strategy aimed at reduction of sputum eosinophils decreases exacerbation rate in patients with asthma. *J Int Med Res.* 2006; 34:129-39.

37. Jayaram L, Pizzichini MM, Cook RJ, Boulet LP, Lemière C, Pizzichini E, et al. Determining asthma treatment by monitoring sputum cell counts: effect on exacerbations. *Eur Respir J.* 2006;27:483-94.

38. Petsky HL, Kynaston JA, Turner C, Li AM, Cates CJ, Lasserson TJ, et al. Tailored interventions based on sputum eosinophils versus clinical symptoms for asthma in children and adults. *Cochrane Database Syst Rev.* 2007;CD005603.

39. Petsky HL, Cates CJ, Lasserson TJ, Li AM, Turner C, Kynaston JA, et al. A systematic review and meta-analysis: tailoring asthma treatment on eosinophilic markers (exhaled nitric oxide or sputum eosinophils). *Thorax.* 2012;67:199-208.

40. Flood-Page P, Swenson C, Faiferman I, Matthews J, Williams M, Brannick L, et al. A study to evaluate safety and efficacy of mepolizumab in patients with moderate persistent asthma. *Am J Respir Crit Care Med.* 2007;176:1062-71.

41. Haldar P, Brightling CE, Hargadon B, Gupta S, Monteiro W, Sousa A, et al. Mepolizumab and exacerbations of refractory eosinophilic asthma. *N Engl J Med.* 2009;360:973-84.

42. Nair P, Pizzichini MM, Kjarsgaard M, Inman MD, Efthimiadis A, Pizzichini E, et al. Mepolizumab for prednisone-dependent asthma with sputum eosinophilia. *N Engl J Med.* 2009;360:985-93.

43. Wenzel S, Wilbraham D, Fuller R, Getz EB, Longphre M. Effect of an interleukin-4 variant on late phase asthmatic response to allergen challenge in asthmatic patients: results of two phase 2a studies. *Lancet.* 2007;370:1422-31.

44. Corren J, Busse W, Meltzer EO, Mansfield L, Bensch G, Fahrenholz J, et al. A randomized, controlled, phase 2 study of AMG 317, an IL-4Ralpha antagonist, in patients with asthma. *Am J Respir Crit Care Med.* 2010;181:788-96.

45. Rodrigo GJ, Neffen H, Castro-Rodriguez JA. Efficacy and safety of subcutaneous omalizumab vs placebo as add-on therapy to corticosteroids for children and adults with asthma: a systematic review. *Chest.* 2011;139:28-35.

46. Walker S, Monteil M, Phelan K, Lasserson TJ, Walters EH. Anti-IgE for chronic asthma in adults and children. *Cochrane Database Syst Rev.* 2006;CD003559.

47. van den Berge M, Pauw RG, de Monchy JG, van Minnen CA, Postma DS, Kerstjens HA. Beneficial effects of treatment with anti-IgE antibodies (Omalizumab) in a patient with severe asthma and negative skin-prick test results. *Chest.* 2011;139:190-3.

48. Denning DW, Van Wye J, Lewiston NJ, Stevens DA. Adjunctive therapy of allergic bronchopulmonary aspergillosis with itraconazole. *Chest.* 1991;100:813-9.

49. Stevens DA, Schwartz HJ, Lee JY, Moskovitz BL, Jerome DC, Catanzaro A, et al. A randomised trial of itraconazole in allergic bronchopulmonary aspergillosis. *N Engl J Med.* 2000;342:756-62.

50. Wark PA, Hensley MJ, Saltos N, Boyle MJ, Toneguzzi RC, Epid GD, et al. Anti-inflammatory effect of itraconazole in stable allergic bronchopulmonary aspergillosis: a randomized controlled trial. *J Allergy Clin Immunol.* 2003;111:952-7.

51. Denning DW, O'Driscoll BR, Hogaboam CM, Bowyer P, Niven RM. The link between fungi and severe asthma: a summary of the evidence. *Eur Respir J.* 2006;27:615-26.

52. Denning DW, O'Driscoll BR, Powell G, Chew F, Atherton GT, Vyas A, et al. Randomized controlled trial of oral antifungal treatment for severe asthma with fungal sensitisation. The Fungal Asthma Sensitization Trial (FAST) study. *Am J Respir Crit Care Med.* 2009; 179:11-8.

53. Crosbie PA, Woodhead MA. Long-term macrolide therapy in chronic inflammatory airway diseases. *Eur Respir J.* 2009;33:171-81.

54. Kudoh S, Azuma A, Yamamoto M, Izumi T, Ando M. Improvement of survival in patients with diffuse panbronchiolitis treated with low-dose erythromycin. *Am J Respir Crit Care Med.* 1998;157:1829-32.

55. Richeldi L, Ferrara G, Fabbri LM, Lasserson TJ, Gibson PG. Macrolides for chronic asthma. *Cochrane Database Syst Rev.* 2005;CD002997.

56. Simpson JL, Powell H, Boyle MJ, Scott RJ, Gibson PG. Clarithromycin targets neutrophilic airway inflammation in refractory asthma. *Am J Respir Crit Care Med.* 2008;177:148-55.

57. Benayoun L, Druilhe A, Dombret MC, Aubier M, Pretolani M. Airway structural alterations selectively associated with severe asthma. *Am J Respir Crit Care Med.* 2003;167: 1360-8.

58. Kariyawasam HH, Robinson DS. The role of eosinophils in airway tissue remodelling in asthma. *Curr Opin Immunol.* 2007;19:681-6.

59. Holgate ST. Epithelium dysfunction in asthma. *J Allergy Clin Immunol.* 2007;120: 1233-44.

60. Carroll N, Elliot J, Morton A, James A. The structure of large and small airways in nonfatal and fatal asthma. *Am Rev Respir Dis.* 1993;147:405-10.

61. Siddiqui S, Gupta S, Cruse G, Haldar P, Entwisle J, Mcdonald S, et al. Airway wall geometry in asthma and nonasthmatic eosinophilic bronchitis. *Allergy.* 2009;64:951-8.

62. Gupta S, Raj V, Castro M, Brightling CE. Imaging in severe asthma. *European Respiratory Society Monograph.* 2011;51:160-81.

63. Gupta S, Siddiqui S, Haldar P, Entwisle JJ, Mawby D, Wardlaw AJ, et al. Quantitative analysis of high-resolution computed tomography scans in severe asthma subphenotypes. *Thorax.* 2010;65:775-81.

64. ten Brinke A, Sterk PJ, Masclee AA, Spinhoven P, Schmidt JT, Zwinderman AH, et al. Risk factors of frequent exacerbations in difficult-to-treat asthma. *Eur Respir J.* 2005; 26:812-8.

65. ten Brinke A, Zwinderman AH, Sterk PJ, Rabe KF, Bel EH. Factors associated with persistent airflow limitation in severe asthma. *Am J Respir Crit Care Med.* 2001;164:744-8.

66. Burrowes KS, Swan AJ, Warren NJ, Tawhai MH. Towards a virtual lung: multi-scale, multi-physics modelling of the pulmonary system. *Philos Transact A Math Phys Eng Sci.* 2008;366:3247-63.

67. Lin CL, Tawhai MH, McLennan G, Hoffman EA. Computational fluid dynamics. *IEEE Eng Med Biol Mag.* 2009;28:25-33.

68. Brook BS, Peel SE, Hall IP, Politi AZ, Sneyd J, Bai Y, et al. A biomechanical model of agonist-initiated contraction in the asthmatic airway. *Respir Physiol Neurobiol.* 2010; 170:4458.

Novel Treatment Strategies in Refractory Asthma

Neil C Thomson, Rekha Chaudhuri

CURRENT MANAGEMENT OF REFRACTORY ASTHMA

A majority of adults with asthma have mild or moderate disease that can be controlled by inhaled corticosteroids (ICS) alone or in combination with inhaled long-acting β_2-agonist (LABA) bronchodilators.[1] Five to ten percent of patients have more severe asthma and often, despite maximal drug treatment, experience considerable morbidity, and generate high healthcare costs. Systematic evaluation should be undertaken to distinguish patients with refractory or treatment resistant asthma from those with 'difficult-to-treat' asthma due to poor adherence, persistent allergen exposure, untreated comorbidities, dysfunctional breathing, or psychological problems.[2,3] The British Guidelines on the Management of Asthma,[4] US Expert Panel Report 3 (EPR-3),[5] and International Global Initiative for Asthma (GINA) guidelines[1] have similar recommendations on the management of chronic asthma, with stepwise treatment aimed at controlling symptoms. Steps 4 and 5 of the British and GINA guidelines and steps 4–6 of the EPR-3 guidelines reflect the stage at which asthma is considered severe or refractory. Step 4 of the British and GINA guidelines and step 5 of the ERP-3 guidelines advise high-dose ICS along with trials of leukotriene receptor antagonists and theophyllines and at the highest step of treatment, daily oral corticosteroids are added.

Omalizumab, a humanized monoclonal antibody reduces free IgE by almost 95%, by binding to the C_H3 region on IgE and blocks it binding to its specific high-affinity receptor.[6] Over 50% of patients with severe asthma have allergic IgE-mediated asthma,[7] and omalizumab is a therapeutic option for those patients with serum IgE levels in the range of 30–1500 IU/mL. Anti-IgE therapy is recommended by the British[4] and GINA[1] guidelines for patients at step 5 and by the EPR-3 guidelines at steps 5 and 6.[5] Due to the high cost of this treatment, different countries have specific criteria to maximize benefit in selected populations of patients. A Cochrane review concluded that the addition of omalizumab to usual therapy is effective in moderate-to-severe allergic asthma with a significant reduction in ICS and rescue medication dose, but no reduction in exacerbations in patients with severe asthma requiring oral corticosteroids.[8] In a recent systematic review of eight clinical trials that included 3,429 participants,[9] omalizumab decreased the risk of asthma exacerbations at the end of stable (RR 0.57, 95% CI: 0.48–0.66) and adjustable corticosteroid phases (RR 0.55, 95% CI: 0.47–0.64). At the end of the corticosteroid reduction phase, subjects treated with omalizumab were more likely to withdraw from corticosteroids completely compared to placebo. The safety profile of omalizumab has been analyzed from clinical trials of over 7,500 patients and by postmarketing safety data on 57,300 patients and has been shown to be favorable.[10] The incidence of anaphylaxis was 0.14% in omalizumab treated patients and 0.07% in control patients in clinical trials and 0.2% in the postmarketing data.[10] Serious adverse effects were similar in omalizumab (3.8%) and placebo groups (5.3%).[9] Anaphylactic reaction risk was 0.33% in omalizumab groups compared to 0.24% in placebo groups.[9] The FDA recently raised concerns about the cardiovascular and cerebrovascular safety of omalizumab based on preliminary data from a five-year epidemiological study designed to evaluate clinical effectiveness and long-term safety in approximately 5,000 patients with moderate-to-severe asthma (EXELS).[11] The EXELS study is due to report in its final results in 2012.

The role of immunomodulating corticosteroid-sparing drugs at the highest step of treatment is limited, as there is marked variability in efficacy, significant adverse effects during treatment and no persistence of benefit after stopping treatment.[4] The British guideline suggests a three-month trial of drugs, such as methotrexate, cyclosporine, and gold, after all other drug treatment has proved unsuccessful, and with careful monitoring of treatment effects. The EPR-3 guideline does not support their use and the GINA guideline states that these medications should only be used in selected patients, as their potential corticosteroid-sparing effects may not outweigh the risk of serious adverse effects.

Despite instituting guideline recommendations for the management of severe asthma, a considerable proportion of patients continue to have poorly controlled disease. There is a need for new therapies for this group.[3,12] This chapter will review unlicensed or recently licensed novel treatment strategies for refractory or treatment-resistant asthma.

NOVEL BRONCHODILATORS AND CORTICOSTEROIDS

Refinements in the pharmacological properties of drugs currently used to treat asthma, such as LABAs and ICS is a major focus of drug development.

Ultra-long-acting Bronchodilators

Inhaled ultra-long-acting β_2-agonists (ultra-LABAs), such as indacaterol and carmoterol have bronchodilator effects lasting over 24 hours and are suitable for once daily dosing.[13,14] New inhaled long-acting antimuscarinic (LAMAs) agents, such as aclidinium and NVA-237, which can also be used once daily, may have a role in the treatment of severe asthma, particularly when associated with persistent airflow obstruction.[15] Compounds with dual actions at the β_2-adrenergic receptor and muscarinic receptor, M3 antagonist-beta$_2$-agonist (MABA) bronchodilators are also under development.[14] A number of ultra-LABAs and ICS are being assessed for use as fixed combination inhalers. The once daily administration of ultralong-acting bronchodilators alone or in combination with an ICS should be more convenient for patients and possibly may improve adherence. It is not clear whether these new drugs will be more effective than current long-acting bronchodilators in the treatment of refractory asthma.

Dissociated Corticosteroids

The clinical effects of corticosteroids in asthma are thought to be due mainly to transrepression of proinflammatory transcription factors and to a much lesser extent to transactivation of anti-inflammatory genes. Transactivation is thought to account for the adverse effects of corticosteroids. To improve the therapeutic ratio of corticosteroids, compounds have been developed that dissociate transactivation from transrepression functions.[16] Nonsteroidal selective glucocorticoid receptor modulators (SGRMs), such as ZK 245186 and mapracorat are in development and show promise when tested in experimental systems *in vitro*.[17-19] Several issues remain regarding the effectiveness of these drugs, since certain adverse effects of corticosteroids, such as osteoporosis involves both transactivation and transrepression and some immuneregulatory genes are regulated by transactivation.

BIOLOGICAL AGENTS

A number of biological agents are under development that target cytokines thought to play an important role in the pathogenesis of asthma.

Tumor Necrosis Factor-α Blockers

Tumor necrosis factor-α (TNF-α) is an important cytokine in the innate immune system, and in severe refractory asthma, is thought to promote airway inflammation, airway hyper-responsiveness, as well as play a role in airway modeling.[20] Early studies with the soluble TNF-α receptor blocker, etanercept, in small numbers of subjects, raised expectations by showing improvements in airway hyper-responsiveness, lung function, and quality of life,[21,22] although these findings were not reproduced by others,[23] The results of two large studies using the monoclonal antibodies, golimumab[24] and etanercept[25] have been disappointing. In the first study,[24] 309 patients with severe persistent asthma received golimumab for 24 weeks without showing evidence of efficacy. The study was prematurely terminated, because of the serious adverse effects of severe infections and solid organ malignancies. Post hoc analysis of subgroups revealed that those with onset of asthma after the age of 12 years and those with greater bronchodilator reversibility were more responsive to TNF-α blockade. The second study[25] compared 12 weeks of etanercept with placebo in 132 subjects with moderate-to-severe asthma and found no clinical efficacy, although the drug was well tolerated. Subgroups of patients with refractory asthma may respond to TNF-α blockers,[22,24] but these agents are unlikely to be developed further, because of their poor risk-benefit ratio.[24]

Interleukin-5 Blockers

A persistently raised airway eosinophil count, which is associated with exacerbations,[26,27] is found in a subgroup of adults with poorly controlled severe asthma despite apparently taking adequate doses of corticosteroids. The recognition that IL-5 is a major driver for the production of eosinophils led to the development of a monoclonal antibody against IL-5 or its receptor as a potential therapy for asthma. Initial studies using IL-5 blocker, mepolizumab, demonstrated reductions in blood, and airway eosinophil counts after allergen challenge or after three months of chronic dosing of patients with mild-to-moderate asthma, but failed to show any improvements in symptoms, lung function, or airway hyper-responsiveness.[28,29] Two recent studies in patients with severe asthma, who had a persistent sputum eosinophilia, despite inhaled or oral corticosteroid treatment, demonstrated a decrease in exacerbation rates with longer-term treatment with mepolizumab, which was associated with reductions in blood and sputum eosinophil numbers.[30,31] One of these studies, which was a small trial in 20 patients with severe asthma receiving chronic oral prednisone therapy, reported a significant prednisone sparing effect of 84% of the maximum possible dose in the 9 patients who received five monthly infusions of mepolizumab compared to 48% in the 11 patients who received placebo.[30] The second study in 61 patients who had refractory eosinophilic asthma and a history of recurrent severe exacerbations reported that mepolizumab was associated with fewer severe exacerbations than placebo over the course of treatment for one year (2.0 mepolizumab vs. 3.4 placebo mean exacerbations per subject), although active treatment did not improve symptoms, forced expiratory volume in 1 second (FEV_1), or airway hyper-responsiveness[31] (Figure 11-1). Further studies of the efficacy and safety of mepolizumab and benralizumab (MEDI-563), an IL-5 receptor monoclonal antibody, are underway in larger populations of patients with severe asthma. The potential impact of IL-5 blockers in the treatment of severe asthma is not certain, since the numbers of patients who fulfill the highly specific criteria for treatment may be small.[32]

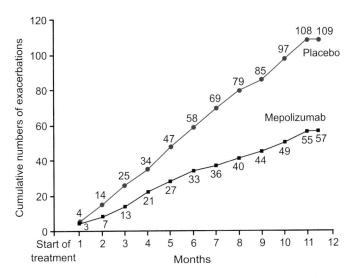

Figure 11-1 Cumulative number of severe exacerbations in each study group over the course of 50 weeks treatment with mepolizumab or placebo. Mean number of exacerbations per subject over the course of the 50-week treatment period was 2.0 in the mepolizumab group as compared to 3.4 in the placebo group (RR, 0.57; 95% CI: 0.32–0.92; p = 0.02). *From* Haldar P, Brightling CE, Hargadon B, Gupta S, Monteiro W, Sousa A, et al. Mepolizumab and exacerbations of refractory eosinophilic asthma. *N Engl J Med.* 2009;360:973-84; *with permission.*

Interleukin-4 and Interleukin-13 Blockers

IL-4 and IL-13, expressed by Th2 cells, are thought to be pivotal cytokines in asthma and are important targets for treatment.[33] IL-13 in particular, is involved in mucous hypersecretion, IgE synthesis regulation, eosinophilic infiltration, and subepithelial fibrosis.[34] Both cytokines share the same receptor system. There is considerable interest in the development of compounds that block IL-4 and IL-13. A humanized soluble IL-4 receptor (altrakincept) and a humanized antibody against IL-4Rα (pascolizumab) showed minimal clinical efficacy.[35] A human anti-IL-13 monoclonal antibody that specifically binds and neutralizes IL-13 (tralokinumab; CAT-354) has a good safety profile[36] and the results of phase II studies are awaited. IMA-638 and IMA-026 are fully humanized IgG1 antibodies that neutralize IL-13 bioactivity. Administration of IMA-026 to 56 patients with mild asthma had no significant inhibitory effect on allergen-induced bronchoconstriction,[37] but IMA-638 did reduce both the early and late allergen-induced responses.[37] Treatment with a dual IL-4 and IL-13 blocker, pitrakinra (Aerovant), which inhibits binding of IL-4 and IL-13 to IL-4Rα receptor complexes, reduces allergen-induced late responses with very few adverse events.[38] Results from a larger study with a dry powder formulation are awaited. Another IL-4Rα antagonist, AMG 317, which is a fully human monoclonal antibody that blocks both IL-4 and IL-13 pathways, was recently studied in 294 subjects with moderate-to-severe asthma.[39] Overall, there was no clinical efficacy, but in the subgroup with higher baseline asthma control questionnaire scores, there was improvement in some clinical outcomes. AIR645, an inhaled oligonucleotide that targets the mRNA that encodes the α-subunit of the human IL-4 receptor is well tolerated in phase I studies[40] and results of a phase II study are awaited. It is likely that a clearer picture of the role of IL-4 and IL-13 blockers in the treatment of severe asthma will emerge over the next 5 years.

Other Interleukin Blockers

Blockers of several other proinflammatory cytokines, such as IL-2,[41] IL-9, IL-17[42] may have a role in the treatment of severe asthma.

Anti-inflammatory Cytokines

The majority of asthma exacerbations are caused by respiratory rhinovirus infections.[43] Patients with asthma may be more susceptible to respiratory viruses because of increased Th2 immunity or impaired Th1 or IL-10 immunity.[44] One approach to the management of exacerbation may be through immunological augmentation with interferons at the time of the exacerbation[43] and inhaled IFN-β is currently under assessment. Alternative approaches to managing or preventing viral-induced exacerbations include the use of specific antiviral therapies and potentially by the development of rhinovirus vaccines.[45] IL-10 has anti-inflammatory properties and may be of potential use for the treatment of severe asthma.

ARACHIDONIC ACID PATHWAY BLOCKERS

Phospholipase Blockers

Phospholipase A2 (PLA2) mobilizes arachidonic acid from membrane phospholipids, which is the first step to the generation of leukotrienes (LT), prostaglandins (PG), and other mediators. There are four types of PLA2, including secretory sPLA2 and cytosolic cPLA2.[46] Several sPLA2 inhibitors[47,48] and cPLA2 inhibitors[49,50] are under investigation. The inhibition of cPLA2α activity affects many allergen-dependent, asthma-associated genes expressed in peripheral blood monocytes to a profile closely resembling that of healthy volunteers.[51] Cytosolic PLA2α blockers may have a potential role in the treatment of severe asthma,[52] because of their inhibitory effects on inflammatory mediator production via both 5-lipoxygenase (LO) and cyclooxygenase pathways.

Leukotriene Modifiers

The cysteinyl leukotrienes, LTC4, LTD4 and LTE4 are synthesized from arachidonic acid by 5-LO and 5-lipoxygenase-activating protein (FLAP) in inflammatory cells, such as eosinophils, alveolar macrophages, and mast cells. Leukotriene synthesis is blocked by inhibition of either 5-LO or 5-FLAP. In addition to inhibiting the production of the cysteinyl LTs, the 5-LO inhibitors, such as zileuton also prevent the formation of LTB4 and other 5-LO products. Several FLAP inhibitors were developed in the 1990s and more recent compounds, such as GSK-2190915 are being assessed in asthma.[53] A selective LTA4 hydrolase inhibitor JNJ-26993135, targeted at reducing LTB4 levels in inflammatory diseases, is undergoing preclinical evaluation.[54,55] A potential advantage of 5-LO inhibitors, FLAP inhibitors, or selective LTA4 hydrolase inhibitors compared to LT-receptor antagonists is the potential efficacy of these drugs in treating severe neutrophilic asthma due to reduced synthesis of the neutrophil chemotactic mediator, LTB4. Several LTB4-receptor antagonists have been synthesized, including LY-293111[56] and SB225002, but none is so far licensed for the treatment of asthma.

Prostaglandin D2 Blockers

Prostaglandin (PG)D2 activates the chemoattractant receptor-homologous molecule expressed on Th2 cells, (CRTH2 receptor) also called the DP2 receptor. PGD2 is released from mast cells as well as other inflammatory cells, including eosinophils, Th2 cells, and macrophages and has proinflammatory effects on a wide range of inflammatory cells. There is considerable interest by the pharmaceutical industry in developing CRTH2 receptor antagonists.[57] Elevated bronchoalveolar lavage concentrations of PGD2 are reported in severe asthma suggesting that CRTH2 receptor antagonists may show particular efficacy in this group.[58]

OTHER DRUG THERAPIES

A number of drugs licensed for conditions other than asthma as well as novel compounds under development may have a role in the management of refractory asthma.

Macrolides

The identification that macrolides have anti-inflammatory effects has generated interest in their use as a treatment for chronic asthma. Early clinical trials in asthma had variable results, with little change in FEV_1 or asthma quality of life, but some improvement in bronchial hyper-responsiveness to methacholine.[59,60] In 2005, a Cochrane systematic review concluded that there was insufficient evidence of benefit to warrant the use of macrolides in chronic asthma;[61] a view reiterated in the British and EPR-3 guidelines.[4,5] Subsequent studies in asthma have reported improvements in symptom scores with azithromycin[62] and quality of life with clarithromycin.[63] Recent studies have tended to focus on the effect of macrolide treatment in subphenotypes of asthma. In one study, an improvement in FEV_1

with clarithromycin was only seen in those subjects who were positive for either *M. pneumoniae* or *C. pneumoniae*, detected by sensitive polymerase chain reaction (PCR) for microbial DNA in nasal and oropharyngeal specimens.[64] These findings were not confirmed in a recent study of 92 mild-to-moderate subjects with asthma in whom bronchial biopsy samples were used to stratify with PCR positivity to these two organisms.[65] In the study 12 weeks treatment with clarithromycin produced no improvement in lung function or asthma control. There was a reduction in bronchial hyper-responsiveness to methacholine in PCR-negative, but not PCR-positive subjects, implying that stratification based on antibacterial effects is not useful in identifying responders. The anti-inflammatory effects of macrolides on neutrophils may help identify likely responders. However, although a reduction in sputum neutrophils and IL-8 levels with clarithromycin was reported in patients with neutrophilic asthma, there was no improvement in lung function or asthma control.[63]

The prevalence of serious adverse effects of long-term treatment with macrolides is low,[66-69] although there is the potential for microbial resistance. For example, with long-term azithromycin use in cystic fibrosis, erythromycin resistance to *Staphylococcus aureus* increased from 6.9 to 53.8%, and clarithromycin resistance to *Haemophilus* sp. from 3.7 to 37.5%.[70] The recent development of chemically modified nonantibiotic macrolides that maintain anti-inflammatory properties may overcome the risk of drug resistant microbial organisms associated with long-term macrolide therapy. Further work is needed to determine whether there is a place for macrolides in the treatment of asthma.

Antifungal Therapy

Chronic allergic bronchopulmonary aspergillosis (ABPA) occurs in a small proportion of patients with severe asthma and can lead to the development of proximal bronchiectasis and pulmonary fibrosis. The criteria used to diagnose chronic APBA are not universally agreed upon, but usually include specific IgE sensitization to *Aspergillus fumigatus* and colonization of the airways with this fungus. These criteria are often accompanied by an elevated serum IgG to *Aspergillus fumigatus,* a raised peripheral blood eosinophil count, a raised total serum IgE level >1,000 IU/mL, and fixed or transient chest radiographic infiltrates. Corticosteroids are the mainstay of treatment and in some cases supplemented by antifungal therapy. Two randomized controlled trials using itraconazole for 16 weeks in asthmatics with APBA demonstrated modest reductions in oral corticosteroid dose or exacerbation rates and decreases in sputum eosinophil and total serum IgE levels.[71-73] A clinical entity categorized as severe asthma with fungal sensitization (SAFS) has recently been described.[74] These individuals are immunologically sensitized to at least 1 of 7 fungi and have a total serum IgE level <1,000 IU/mL and negative precipitins to

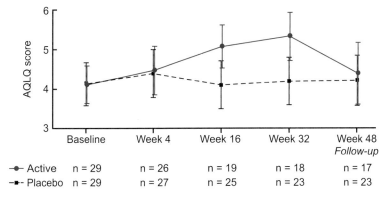

Figure 11-2 Changes in Asthma Quality of Life Questionnaire (AQLQ) by time on study. Numbers of subjects studied are listed below each time point, and 95% confidence intervals (CI) are shown. Higher scores indicate improvement. The change at 32 weeks was +0.85 (95% CI: 0.28, 1.41) in the antifungal therapy group and –0.01 (95% CI: –0.43, 0.42) in the placebo group. *From* Denning DW, O'Driscoll BR, Powell G, Chew F, Atherton GT, Vyas A, et al. Randomized controlled trial of oral antifungal treatment for severe asthma with fungal sensitization: The Fungal Asthma Sensitization Trial (FAST) study. *Am J Respir Crit Care Med.* 2009;179:11-8; *with permission.*

Aspergillus fumigatus. Fifty-eight patients with SAFS were treated in a randomized controlled study with oral itraconazole 400 mg daily or placebo for 32 weeks.[75] At 32 weeks, the improvement in Asthma Quality of Life Questionnaire (AQLQ) score was significantly greater in the antifungal group, compared with placebo (+0.85 vs. 0.01) (Figure 11-2). There are several case reports of adrenal suppression occurring with ICS and itraconazole,[76,77] which may limit the widespread long-term use of itraconazole.

Phosphodiesterase-4 Inhibitors

The phosphodiesterase (PDE)-4 inhibitors, cilomilast and roflumilast, have immuno-modulatory activity over a number of inflammatory cells, potentially relevant to the treatment of severe asthma.[78] Clinical trials with cilomilast in asthma did not show benefit whereas clinical improvements are reported with roflumilast.[78-82] In a dose range and efficacy study, in mild-to-moderate asthma, roflumilast increased lung function, particularly at the highest doses used.[81] The use of high doses of roflumilast in refractory asthma to improve lung function may be limited by gastrointestinal side effects. Inhaled PDE4 inhibitors have the potential to improve the therapeutic index of these agents.[83,84]

Protein Kinase Inhibitors

The use of small molecules to inhibit different protein kinases involved in cellular signaling of proinflammatory cytokines has been investigated in chronic inflammatory diseases.[85,86] p38 mitogen-activated protein kinase (MAPK) inhibitors target downstream signaling pathways whereas more upstream pathways can be blocked with spleen tyrosine kinase (SYK) inhibitors or janus kinase (JAKs) inhibitors.[85] In addition to potentially reducing proinflammatory cytokines in severe asthma, p38MAPK inhibition may help reverse corticosteroid insensitivity.[87] To reduce systemic adverse effects, inhaled formulations of these inhibitors are under development.[88] A phase III study evaluating masitinib, a tyrosine kinase inhibitor of the c-KIT receptor, in the treatment of severe asthma commenced in early 2011. Preclinical data suggest that phosphoinositide-3-kinase-delta inhibitors could potentially reverse corticosteroid insensitivity in severe asthma.[89] Other protein kinases that are potential targets for inhibition include sphingosine 1-phosphate kinase and rho-kinase.[86,90,91]

Peroxisome Proliferator-activated Receptor-γ Agonists

Peroxisome proliferator-activated receptor-γ (PPARγ) agonists exert anti-inflammatory effects on multiple inflammatory cell types, including eosinophilic and neutrophilic infiltration of the lungs of experimental animals.[92] A pilot study using the PPARγ agonist, rosiglitazone, demonstrated bronchodilator effects in mild-to-moderate smokers with asthma.[93] Clinical trials of the oral PPARγ agonist pioglitazone in severe asthma are underway. The adverse-effect profile of oral rosiglitazone may preclude its development for asthma, although inhaled analogs may overcome such concerns.[90]

Chemokine Antagonists

Chemokines are implicated in inflammatory responses in the lung. CXCR2, the receptor for the chemoattractant cytokine CXCL8, has a role in neutrophil chemotaxis and may be involved in contractile responses of airway smooth muscle in chronic asthma.[94] Clinical trials are underway to evaluate the potential of CXCR2 antagonists for the treatment of asthma.

Endothelin Antagonists

The small peptide endothelin causes bronchoconstriction and has been implicated in contributing to airway remodeling in asthma.[95,96] A clinical trial of the effects of 12 months treatment with the endothelin receptor antagonist sitaxsentan on airway remodeling is underway in patients with severe asthma.

Vitamin D

Stimulation of vitamin D receptors may have an immunomodulatory role in the treatment of refractory asthma.[97] In adult nonsmokers with asthma, reduced vitamin D levels are associated with decreased corticosteroid sensitivity of peripheral blood mononuclear cells.[98] Peripheral blood CD4+ T cells isolated from subjects with corticosteroid-resistant asthma regain sensitivity to corticosteroids following a short course of oral vitamin D.[99] Possibly, supplementation with vitamin D may overcome corticosteroid insensitivity in severe asthma.[97]

Statins

Despite preclinical data showing that statins have pleiotropic anti-inflammatory effects potentially relevant to the treatment of asthma,[100-106] no improvement in symptoms or lung function was found in nonsmokers[107-109] or smokers with mild-to-moderate asthma[110] after short-term treatment. Interestingly, the latter study showed improvements in asthma quality of life.[110] Statins inhibit human airway smooth muscle cell proliferation and it is possible that long-term administration of statins might improve airway remodeling in severe asthma.

BRONCHIAL THERMOPLASTY

Bronchial thermoplasty to the airways is a new treatment technique that involves the delivery of radiofrequency energy to the airways with the aim of reducing airway smooth muscle mass and responsiveness in asthma.[111] Preclinical studies in experimental animals show that bronchial thermoplasty reduces airway smooth muscle,[112] increases airway size,[113,114] and decreases airway responsiveness to methacholine.[112-114] Taken together, these studies support the concept that reducing the amount of functional smooth muscle with bronchial thermoplasty may have a beneficial effect in the treatment of asthma. The 'Alair' bronchial thermoplasty system consists of a small radiofrequency generator and single use catheters in which an expandable electrode array is deployed by a handle mechanism. Bronchial thermoplasty is delivered to patients with asthma by flexible bronchoscopy under moderate sedation over three outpatient sessions.[115]

Efficacy of Bronchial Thermoplasty

In an observational study designed to determine the safety of bronchial thermoplasty in 16 subjects with mild-to-moderate asthma, the intervention resulted in improvements in symptom-free days, morning PEF at 3 months, and a reduction in airway hyper-responsiveness to methacholine that lasted for at least 2 years.[116] In the first randomized controlled study to assess the effects of bronchial thermoplasty, the Asthma Intervention Research (AIR)1 trial,[117] 112 adults with moderate or severe asthma were randomized to receive bronchial thermoplasty or to a control group continuing standard asthma medication. There was a period of abstinence from a long-acting bronchodilator at baseline and after 3, 6, and 12 months. In the bronchial thermoplasty group compared to the control group, the mean rate of mild exacerbations compared to baseline was significantly reduced and there were improvements at 12 months in morning PEF, AQLQ, and ACQ scores. A further randomized controlled study, the Research in Severe Asthma (RISA) trial, assessed the safety of bronchial thermoplasty in 34 patients with more severe disease, half of

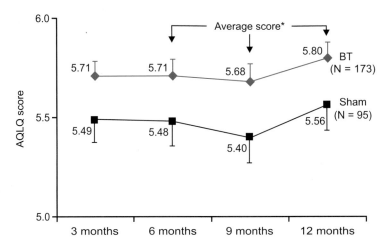

Figure 11-3 Change in Asthma Quality of Life Questionnaire (AQLQ) score over 12 months after treatment with bronchial thermoplasty (BT) (*diamonds*) or sham control (*squares*) in the per protocol population. *Posterior probability of superiority = 97.9%. *From* Castro M, Rubin AS, Laviolette M, Fiterman J, De Andrade Lima M, Shah PL, et al. Effectiveness and safety of bronchial thermoplasty in the treatment of severe asthma: a multicenter, randomized, double-blind, sham-controlled clinical trial. *Am J Respir Crit Care Med.* 2010;181:116-24; *with permission.*

whom were receiving chronic oral corticosteroid therapy in addition to high doses of ICS.[118] Bronchial thermoplasty resulted in significant improvements in ACQ scores and rescue medication use at 22 and 52 weeks after treatment and an improvement in FEV_1 at 22 weeks post-treatment. The efficacy and safety of bronchial thermoplasty has most recently been assessed in a placebo-controlled trial, the AIR2 trial, involving the use of bronchoscopy with sham bronchial thermoplasty in 288 adult subjects with severe asthma.[119] Bronchial thermoplasty resulted in improvements from baseline in AQLQ scores compared with sham (bronchial thermoplasty, 1.35 vs. sham, 1.16), with 79% of bronchial thermoplasty and 64% of sham subjects achieved changes in AQLQ of 0.5 or greater (Figure 11-3). In the post-treatment period, the bronchial thermoplasty group experienced fewer severe exacerbations, emergency department visits, and days missed from work/school compared with the sham group.

Adverse Effects of Bronchial Thermoplasty

Bronchial thermoplasty is associated with short-term increases in asthma-related morbidity, including increased hospitalizations for asthma. Long-term safety of bronchial thermoplasty in patients recruited to the AIR1 trial reported the absence of clinical complications and the maintenance of stable lung function over a 5-year period postbronchial thermoplasty.[120] Computed tomography scans taken at baseline and annually for 5 years after bronchial thermoplasty in the first 16 subjects with mild-to-moderate asthma who received treatment[116] showed no clinically significant changes in the airways, such as bronchiectasis, parenchymal fibrosis, or airway stenosis.[121]

Place in Management of Refractory Asthma

The procedure has been approved by the American Food and Drug Administration (FDA) for the treatment of severe persistent asthma. Factors that predict a therapeutic response to the bronchial thermoplasty in patients with severe asthma have not been identified from published clinical trials.

IMMUNOTHERAPY

Specific allergen immunotherapy using subcutaneous injections [SCIT] over 3–5 years is recommended in asthma guidelines.[1,4,5] Most clinical trials are in patients with mild-to-moderate asthma[122] and this treatment has a limited role in severe asthma,[122] because of an increased risk of systemic reactions to immunotherapy injections.[123] Modifications to immunotherapy are under investigation,[124] such as combining SCIT with omalizumab pretreatment to reduce systemic allergic reactions.[125]

AVOIDANCE MEASURES

There is very little evidence that avoidance of allergens alters asthma control, especially in those with severe asthma.[1,4,126,127] The EPR-3 guideline recommends that patients should reduce exposure as much as possible to allergens to which they are sensitized and exposed and use multifaceted approaches; humidifiers are not recommended.[5] The addition of domestic mechanical heat recovery ventilation system to house-dust mite eradication strategies over 12 months in 120 adults with asthma and allergic to house-dust mite did not achieve a reduction in mite allergen levels, but did result in modest improvement in evening PEF.[128]

FACTORS INFLUENCING THE RESPONSE TO NOVEL THERAPIES

Both genotypic and phenotypic factors (Table 11-1), either alone or in combination, may influence the response to drug treatment for asthma.[129] The failure of some novel therapies to show efficacy when administered to heterogeneous groups of patients with severe asthma can be overcome by targeting individuals with a responsive phenotype.[22,30,31] The development of novel therapies for severe asthma is likely in the future to involve using a combination of clinical factors and genotypic and/or phenotypic inflammatory biomarkers to identify patients responsive to a specific intervention.

Table 11-1	Genotypic and Phenotypic Factors in Severe Asthma that may Influence the Response to Novel Therapies		
Clinical phenotypes	*Genotypes*	*Inflammatory phenotypes*	
Exacerbation prone[130]	Adrenergic β_2-receptor polymorphisms[137,138]	Eosinophilic[147,148]	
Corticosteroid-resistant asthma[131]		Neutrophilic[147,148]	
Smokers with asthma[90,132]	Polymorphisms of the arachidonic acid pathway[139-143]	Paucigranulocytic[147,148]	
Chronic persistent airflow obstruction[133-135]	Polymorphisms associated with corticosteroid sensitivity[144-146]	Th1 and Th2 cytokine profiles[149]	
Asthma associated with bronchiectasis[136]			
Age of onset	Atopy		

CONCLUSION

Many patients with severe asthma remain symptomatic despite currently available therapies. Despite considerable efforts by the pharmaceutical industry, anti-IgE therapy and bronchial thermoplasty are the only novel treatments that have been licensed over the last 10 years for the treatment of severe asthma. There is an urgent need to identify new therapies that are both effective and safe. Improvements in current molecules as well as a wide range of novel therapies are under different stages of development for the treatment of refractory asthma.

In the future, both genotypic and phenotypic factors, either alone or in combination, are likely to guide the choice of intervention in each individual with severe asthma.

REFERENCES

1. Bateman ED, Hurd SS, Barnes PJ, Bousquet J, Drazen JM, FitzGerald M, et al. Global strategy for asthma management and prevention: GINA executive summary. *Euro Respir J.* 2008;31:143-78.
2. Bel EH, Sousa A, Fleming L, Bush A, Chung KF, Versnel J, et al. Diagnosis and definition of severe refractory asthma: an international consensus statement from the Innovative Medicine Initiative (IMI). *Thorax.* 2011;66:910-7.
3. Chanez P, Wenzel SE, Anderson GP, Anto JM, Bel EH, Boulet LP, et al. Severe asthma in adults: what are the important questions? *J Allergy Clin Immunol.* 2007;119:1337-48.
4. British Thoracic Society Scottish Intercollegiate Guidelines Network. British guideline on the management of asthma. *Thorax.* 2008;63:1-121.
5. National Asthma Education and Prevention Program. Expert Panel Report 3 (EPR-3): Guidelines for the Diagnosis and Management of Asthma-Summary Report 2007. *J Allergy Clin Immunol.* 2007;120:S94-138.
6. Hamelmann E. The rationale for treating allergic asthma with anti-IgE. *Eur Respir Rev.* 2007;16:61-6.
7. The ENFUMOSA cross-sectional European multicentre study of the clinical phenotype of chronic severe asthma. European Network for Understanding Mechanisms of Severe Asthma. *Eur Respir J.* 2003;22:470-7.

8. Walker S, Monteil M, Phelan K, Lasserson TJ, Walters EH. Anti-IgE for chronic asthma in adults and children. *Cochrane Database Syst Rev.* 2006:CD003559.

9. Rodrigo GJ, Neffen H, Castro-Rodriguez JA. Efficacy and safety of subcutaneous omalizumab vs placebo as add-on therapy to corticosteroids for children and adults with asthma: a systematic review. *Chest.* 2011;139:28-35.

10. Corren J, Casale TB, Lanier B, Buhl R, Holgate S, Jimenez P. Safety and tolerability of omalizumab. *Clin Exp Allergy.* 2009;39:788-97.

11. Long AA, Fish JE, Rahmaoui A, Miller MK, Bradley MS, Taki HN, et al. Baseline characteristics of patients enrolled in EXCELS: a cohort study. *Ann Allergy Asthma Immunol.* 2009;103:212-9.

12. Barnes PJ. New therapies for asthma. *Trends Mol Med.* 2006;12:515-20.

13. Cazzola M, Segreti A, Matera MG. Novel bronchodilators in asthma. *Curr Opin Pulm Med.* 2010;16:6-12.

14. Cazzola M, Matera MG. Novel long-acting bronchodilators for COPD and asthma. *Br J Pharmacol.* 2008;155:291-9.

15. Park HW, Yang MS, Park CS, Kim TB, Moon HB, Min KU, et al. Additive role of tiotropium in severe asthmatics and Arg16Gly in ADRB2 as a potential marker to predict response. *Allergy.* 2009;64:778-83.

16. De Bosscher K, Haegeman G, Elewaut D. Targeting inflammation using selective glucocorticoid receptor modulators. *Curr Opin Pharmacol.* 2010;10:497-504.

17. Schäcke H, Schottelius A, Döcke WD, Strehlke P, Jaroch S, Schmees N, et al. Dissociation of transactivation from transrepression by a selective glucocorticoid receptor agonist leads to separation of therapeutic effects from side effects. *Proc Natl Acad Sci U S A.* 2004;101:227-32.

18. Schäcke H, Zollner TM, Döcke WD, Rehwinkel H, Jaroch S, Skuballa W, et al. Characterization of ZK 245186, a novel, selective glucocorticoid receptor agonist for the topical treatment of inflammatory skin diseases. *Br J Pharmacol.* 2009;158:1088-103.

19. Zhang Jin-Zhong, Cavet ME, VanDerMeid KR, Salvador-Silva M, López FJ, Ward KW. BOL-303242-X, a novel selective glucocorticoid receptor agonist, with full anti-inflammatory properties in human ocular cells. *Mol Vis.* 2009;15:2606-16.

20. Brightling C, Berry M, Amrani Y. Targeting TNF-alpha: a novel therapeutic approach for asthma. *J Allergy Clin Immunol.* 2008;121:5-10.

21. Howarth PH, Babu KS, Arshad HS, Lau L, Buckley M, McConnell W, et al. Tumour necrosis factor (TNFalpha) as a novel therapeutic target in symptomatic corticosteroid dependent asthma. *Thorax.* 2005;60:1012-8.

22. Erzurum SC. Inhibition of tumor necrosis factor alpha for refractory asthma. *N Eng J Med.* 2006;354:754-8.

23. Morjaria JB, Chauhan AJ, Babu KS, Polosa R, Davies DE, Holgate ST. The role of a soluble TNF alpha receptor fusion protein (etanercept) in corticosteroid refractory asthma: a double blind, randomised, placebo controlled trial. *Thorax.* 2008;63:584-91.

24. Wenzel SE, Barnes PJ, Bleecker ER, Bousquet J, Busse W, Dahlén SE, et al. A randomized, double-blind, placebo-controlled study of tumor necrosis factor-alpha blockade in severe persistent asthma. *Am J Respir Crit Care Med.* 2009;179:549-58.

25. Holgate ST, Noonan M, Chanez P, Busse W, Dupont L, Pavord I, et al. Efficacy and safety of etanercept in moderate-to-severe asthma: a randomised, controlled trial. *Eur Respir J.* 2011;37:1352-9.

26. Haldar P, Pavord ID, Shaw DE, Berry MA, Thomas M, Brightling CE, et al. Cluster analysis and clinical asthma phenotypes. *Am J Respir Crit Care Med.* 2008;178:218-24.

27. Green RH, Brightling CE, McKenna S, Hargadon B, Parker D, Bradding P, et al. Asthma exacerbations and sputum eosinophil counts: a randomised controlled trial. *Lancet.* 2002;360:1715-21.

28. Leckie MJ, ten Brinke A, Khan J, Diamant Z, O'Connor BJ, Walls CM, et al. Effects of an interleukin-5 blocking monoclonal antibody on eosinophils, airway hyper-responsiveness, and the late asthmatic response. *Lancet.* 2000;356:2144-8.

29. Flood-Page P, Swenson C, Faiferman I, Matthews J, Williams M, Brannick L, et al. A study to evaluate safety and efficacy of mepolizumab in patients with moderate persistent asthma. *Am J Respir Crit Care Med.* 2007;176:1062-71.

30. Nair P, Pizzichini MM, Kjarsgaard M, Inman MD, Efthimiadis A, Pizzichini E, et al. Mepolizumab for prednisone-dependent asthma with sputum eosinophilia. *N Engl J Med.* 2009;360:985-93.

31. Haldar P, Brightling CE, Hargadon B, Gupta S, Monteiro W, Sousa A, et al. Mepolizumab and exacerbations of refractory eosinophilic asthma. *N Engl J Med.* 2009;360:973-84.

32. Wenzel SE. Eosinophils in asthma—closing the loop or opening the door? *N Engl J Med.* 2009;360:1026-8.

33. Oh CK, Geba GP, Molfino N. Investigational therapeutics targeting the IL-4/IL-13/STAT-6 pathway for the treatment of asthma. *Eur Respir Rev.* 2010;19:46-54.

34. Mitchell J, Dimov V, Townley RG. IL-13 and the IL-13 receptor as therapeutic targets for asthma and allergic disease. *Curr Opin Investig Drugs.* 2010;11:527-34.

35. Corren J. Cytokine inhibition in severe asthma: current knowledge and future directions. *Curr Opin Pulm Med.* 2011;17:29-33.

36. Singh D, Kane B, Molfino NA, Faggioni R, Roskos L, Woodcock A. A phase 1 study evaluating the pharmacokinetics, safety and tolerability of repeat dosing with a human IL-13 antibody (CAT-354) in subjects with asthma. *BMC Pulm Med.* 2010;10:3.

37. Gauvreau GM, Boulet L-P, Cockcroft DW, Fitzgerald JM, Carlsten C, Davis BE, et al. The effects of IL-13 blockade on allergen-induced airway responses in mild atopic asthma. *Am J Respir Crit Care Med.* 2010;183:1007-14.

38. Wenzel S, Wilbraham D, Fuller R, Getz EB, Longphre M. Effect of an interleukin-4 variant on late phase asthmatic response to allergen challenge in asthmatic patients: results of two phase 2a studies. *Lancet.* 2007;370:1422-31.

39. Corren J, Busse W, Meltzer EO, Mansfield L, Bensch G, Fahrenholz J, et al. A randomized, controlled, phase 2 study of AMG 317, an IL-4Ralpha antagonist, in patients with asthma. *Am J Respir Crit Care Med.* 2010;181:788-96.

40. Hodges MR, Castelloe E, Chen A, Geary RS, Karras JG, Shapiro D, et al. Randomized, Double-Blind, Placebo Controlled First in Human Study Of Inhaled AIR645, an IL-4Ra Oligonucleotide, in Healthy Volunteers. *Am J Respir Crit Care Med.* 2009;179: A3640.

41. Busse WW, Israel E, Nelson HS, Baker JW, Charous BL, Young DY, et al. Daclizumab improves asthma control in patients with moderate to severe persistent asthma: a randomized, controlled trial. *Am J Respir Crit Care Med.* 2008;178:1002-8.

42. Park SJ, Lee YC. Interleukin-17 regulation: an attractive therapeutic approach for asthma. *Respir Res.* 2010;11:78.

43. Sykes A, Johnston SL. Etiology of asthma exacerbations. *J Allergy Clin Immunol.* 2008; 122:685-8.

44. Message SD, Laza-Stanca V, Mallia P, Parker HL, Zhu J, Kebadze T, et al. Rhinovirus-induced lower respiratory illness is increased in asthma and related to virus load and Th1/2 cytokine and IL-10 production. *Proc Natl Acad Sci U S A.* 2008;105:13562-7.

45. Edlmayr J, Niespodziana K, Popow-Kraupp T, Krzyzanek V, Focke-Tejkl M, Blaas D, et al. Antibodies induced with recombinant VP1 from human rhinovirus exhibit cross-neutralisation. *Eur Respir J.* 2011;37:44-52.

46. Magrioti V, Kokotos G. Phospholipase A2 inhibitors as potential therapeutic agents for the treatment of inflammatory diseases. *Expert Opin Ther Pat.* 2010;20:1-18.

47. Bowton DL, Dmitrienko AA, Israel E, Zeiher BG, Sides GD. Impact of a soluble phospholipase A2 inhibitor on inhaled allergen challenge in subjects with asthma. *J Asthma.* 2005;42:65-71.

48. Lai Y, Oslund RC, Bollinger JG, Henderson WR Jr, Santana LF, Altemeier WA, et al. Eosinophil cysteinyl leukotriene synthesis mediated by exogenous secreted phospholipase A2 group X. *J Biol Chem.* 2010;285:41491-500.

49. Myou S, Sano H, Fujimura M, Zhu X, Kurashima K, Kita T, et al. Blockade of eosinophil migration and airway hyperresponsiveness by cPLA2-inhibition. *Nat Immunol.* 2001; 2:145-9.

50. McKew JC, Lee KL, Shen MW, Thakker P, Foley MA, Behnke ML, et al. Indole cytosolic phospholipase A2 alpha inhibitors: discovery and *in vitro* and *in vivo* characterization of 4-{3-[5-chloro-2-(2-{[(3,4-dichlorobenzyl)sulfonyl]amino}ethyl)-1-(diphenylmethyl)-1H-indol-3-yl]propyl}benzoic acid, efipladib. *J Med Chem.* 2008; 51:3388-413.

51. Whalen KA, Legault H, Hang C, Hill A, Kasaian M, Donaldson D, et al. In vitro allergen challenge of peripheral blood induces differential gene expression in mononuclear cells of asthmatic patients: inhibition of cytosolic phospholipase A2α overcomes the asthma-associated response. *Clin Exp Allergy.* 2008;38:1590-605.

52. Sokolowska M, Stefanska J, Wodz-Naskiewicz K, Cieslak M, Pawliczak R. Cytosolic phospholipase A2 group IVA is overexpressed in patients with persistent asthma and regulated by the promoter microsatellites. *J Allergy Clin Immunol.* 2010;125:1393-5.

53. Evans JF, Ferguson AD, Mosley RT, Hutchinson JH. What's all the FLAP about?: 5-lipoxygenase-activating protein inhibitors for inflammatory diseases. *Trends Pharmacol Sci.* 2008;29:72-8.

54. Rao NL, Dunford PJ, Xue X, Jiang X, Lundeen KA, Coles F, et al. Anti-inflammatory activity of a potent, selective leukotriene A4 hydrolase inhibitor in comparison with the 5-lipoxygenase inhibitor zileuton. *J Pharmacol Exp Ther.* 2007;321:1154-60.

55. Rao NL, Riley JP, Banie H, Xue X, Sun B, Crawford S, et al. Leukotriene A(4) hydrolase inhibition attenuates allergic airway inflammation and hyperresponsiveness. *Am J Respir Crit Care Med.* 2010;181:899-907.

56. Silbaugh SA, Stengel PW, Cockerham SL, Froelich LL, Bendele AM, Spaethe SM, et al. Pharmacologic actions of the second generation leukotriene B4 receptor antagonist LY29311: in vivo pulmonary studies. *Naunyn Schmiedebergs Arch Pharmacol.* 2000;361: 397-404.

57. Schuligoi R, Sturm E, Luschnig P, Konya V, Philipose S, Sedej M, et al. CRTH2 and D-type prostanoid receptor antagonists as novel therapeutic agents for inflammatory diseases. *Pharmacology.* 2010;85:372-82.

58. Balzar S, Fajt ML, Comhair SA, Erzurum SC, Bleecker E, Busse WW, et al. Mast cell phenotype, location, and activation in severe asthma. Data from the Severe Asthma Research Program. *Am J Respir Crit Care Med.* 2011;183:299-309.

59. Amayasu H, Yoshida S, Ebana S, Yamamoto Y, Nishikawa T, Shoji T, et al. Clarithromycin suppresses bronchial hyperresponsiveness associated with eosinophilic inflammation in patients with asthma. *Ann Allergy Asthma Immunol.* 2000;84:594-8.

60. Kostadima E, Tsiodras S, Alexopoulos EI, Kaditis AG, Mavrou I, Georgatou N, et al. Clarithromycin reduces the severity of bronchial hyperresponsiveness in patients with asthma. *Eur Respir J*. 2004;23:714-7.

61. Richeldi L, Ferrara G, Fabbri LM, Lasserson TJ, Gibson PG. Macrolides for chronic asthma. *Cochrane Database Syst Rev*. 2005:CD002997.

62. Hahn DL, Plane MB, Mahdi OS, Byrne GI. Secondary Outcomes of a Pilot Randomized Trial of Azithromycin Treatment for Asthma. *PLoS Clin Trials*. 2006;1:e11.

63. Simpson JL, Powell H, Boyle MJ, Scott RJ, Gibson PG. Clarithromycin targets neutrophilic airway inflammation in refractory asthma. *Am J Respir Crit Care Med*. 2008;177:148-55.

64. Kraft M, Cassell GH, Pak J, Martin RJ. Mycoplasma pneumoniae and Chlamydia pneumoniae in asthma: effect of clarithromycin. *Chest*. 2002;121:1782-8.

65. Sutherland ER, King TS, Icitovic N, Ameredes BT, Bleecker E, Boushey HA, et al. A trial of clarithromycin for the treatment of suboptimally controlled asthma. *J Allergy Clin Immunol*. 2010;126:747-53.

66. Florescu DF, Murphy PJ, Kalil AC. Effects of prolonged use of azithromycin in patients with cystic fibrosis: a meta-analysis. *Pulm Pharmacol Ther*. 2009;22:467-72.

67. Gottlieb J, Szangolies J, Koehnlein T, Golpon H, Simon A, Welte T. Long-term azithromycin for bronchiolitis obliterans syndrome after lung transplantation. *Transplantation*. 2008; 85:36-41.

68. Kadota J, Mukae H, Ishii H, Nagata T, Kaida H, Tomono K, et al. Long-term efficacy and safety of clarithromycin treatment in patients with diffuse panbronchiolitis. *Respir Med*. 2003;97:844-50.

69. Azuma A, Kudoh S. Securing the safety and efficacy of macrolide therapy for chronic small airway diseases. *Inter Med*. 2005;44:167-8.

70. Phaff SJ, Tiddens HA, Verbrugh HA, Ott A. Macrolide resistance of Staphylococcus aureus and Haemophilus species associated with long-term azithromycin use in cystic fibrosis. *J Antimicrob Chemother*. 2006;57:741-6.

71. Stevens DA, Schwartz HJ, Lee JY, Moskovitz BL, Jerome DC, Catanzaro A, et al. A randomized trial of itraconazole in allergic bronchopulmonary aspergillosis. *N Engl J Med*. 2000;342:756-62.

72. Wark PA, Hensley MJ, Saltos N, Boyle MJ, Toneguzzi RC, Epid GD, et al. Anti-inflammatory effect of itraconazole in stable allergic bronchopulmonary aspergillosis: a randomized controlled trial. *J Allergy Clin Immunol*. 2003;111:952-7.

73. Wark PA, Gibson PG, Wilson AJ. Azoles for allergic bronchopulmonary aspergillosis associated with asthma. *Cochrane Database Syst Rev*. 2004:CD001108.

74. Denning DW, O'Driscoll BR, Hogaboam CM, Bowyer P, Niven RM. The link between fungi and severe asthma: a summary of the evidence. *Eur Respir J*. 2006;27:615-26.

75. Denning DW, O'Driscoll BR, Powell G, Chew F, Atherton GT, Vyas A, et al. Randomized controlled trial of oral antifungal treatment for severe asthma with fungal sensitization: The Fungal Asthma Sensitization Trial (FAST) study. *Am J Respir Crit Care Med*. 2009; 179:11-8.

76. Parmar JS, Howell T, Kelly J, Bilton D. Profound adrenal suppression secondary to treatment with low dose inhaled steroids and itraconazole in allergic bronchopulmonary aspergillosis in cystic fibrosis. *Thorax*. 2002;57:749-50.

77. Skov M, Main KM, Sillesen IB, Müller J, Koch C, Lanng S. Iatrogenic adrenal insufficiency as a side-effect of combined treatment of itraconazole and budesonide. *Eur Respir J*. 2002;20:127-33.

78. Lipworth BJ. Phosphodiesterase-4 inhibitors for asthma and chronic obstructive pulmonary disease. *Lancet*. 2005;365:167-75.

79. Calverley PM, Rabe KF, Goehring UM, Kristiansen S, Fabbri LM, Martinez FJ; M2-124 and M2-125 study groups. Roflumilast in symptomatic chronic obstructive pulmonary disease: two randomised clinical trials. *Lancet*. 2009;374:685-94.

80. Fabbri LM, Calverley PM, Izquierdo-Alonso JL, Bundschuh DS, Brose M, Martinez FJ, et al. Roflumilast in moderate-to-severe chronic obstructive pulmonary disease treated with longacting bronchodilators: two randomised clinical trials. *Lancet*. 2009;374:695-703.

81. Bateman ED, Izquierdo JL, Harnest U, Hofbauer P, Magyar P, Schmid-Wirlitsch C, et al. Efficacy and safety of roflumilast in the treatment of asthma. *Ann Allergy Asthma Immunol*. 2006;96:679-86.

82. Bousquet J, Aubier M, Sastre J, Izquierdo JL, Adler LM, Hofbauer P, et al. Comparison of roflumilast, an oral anti-inflammatory, with beclomethasone dipropionate in the treatment of persistent asthma. *Allergy*. 2006;61:72-8.

83. Chapman RW, House A, Richard J, Prelusky D, Lamca J, Wang P, et al. Pharmacology of a potent and selective inhibitor of PDE4 for inhaled administration. *Eur J Pharmacol*. 2010;643:274-81.

84. Singh D, Petavy F, Macdonald AJ, Lazaar AL, O'Connor BJ. The inhaled phosphodiesterase 4 inhibitor GSK256066 reduces allergen challenge responses in asthma. *Respir Res*. 2010; 11:26.

85. Cohen S, Fleischmann R. Kinase inhibitors: a new approach to rheumatoid arthritis treatment. *Curr Opin Rheumatol*. 2010;22:330-5.

86. Hammaker D, Firestein GS. "Go upstream, young man": lessons learned from the p38 saga. *Ann Rheum Dis*. 2010;69:i77-82.

87. Bhavsar P, Khorasani N, Hew M, Johnson M, Chung KF. Effect of p38 MAPK inhibition on corticosteroid suppression of cytokine release in severe asthma. *Eur Respir J*. 2010; 35:750-6.

88. Riccaboni M, Bianchi I, Petrillo P. Spleen tyrosine kinases: biology, therapeutic targets and drugs. *Drug Discov Today*. 2010;15:517-30.

89. Marwick JA, Caramori G, Stevenson CS, Casolari P, Jazrawi E, Barnes PJ, et al. Inhibition of PI3Kdelta restores glucocorticoid function in smoking-induced airway inflammation in mice. *Am J Respir Crit Care Med*. 2009;179:542-8.

90. Spears M, Cameron E, Chaudhuri R, Thomson NC. Challenges of treating asthma in people who smoke. *Expert Rev Clin Immunol*. 2010;6:257-68.

91. Schaafsma D, Gosens R, Zaagsma J, Halayko AJ, Meurs H. Rho kinase inhibitors: a novel therapeutical intervention in asthma? *Eur J Pharmacol*. 2008;585:398-406.

92. Spears M, McSharry C, Thomson NC. Peroxisome proliferator-activated receptor-gamma agonists as potential anti-inflammatory agents in asthma and chronic obstructive pulmonary disease. *Clin Exp Allergy*. 2006;36:1494-504.

93. Spears M, Donnelly I, Jolly L, Brannigan M, Ito K, McSharry C, et al. Bronchodilatory effect of the PPAR-gamma agonist rosiglitazone in smokers with asthma. *Clin Pharmacol Ther*. 2009;86:49-53.

94. Chapman RW, Phillips JE, Hipkin RW, Curran AK, Lundell D, Fine JS. CXCR2 antagonists for the treatment of pulmonary disease. *Pharmacol Ther*. 2009;121:55-68.

95. Pégorier S, Arouche N, Dombret MC, Aubier M, Pretolani M. Augmented epithelial endothelin-1 expression in refractory asthma. *J Allergy Clin Immunol*. 2007;120:1301-7.

96. McWhinnie R, Pechkovsky DV, Zhou D, Lane D, Halayko AJ, Knight DA, et al. Endothelin-1 induces hypertrophy and inhibits apoptosis in human airway smooth muscle cells. *Am J Physiol Lung Cell Mol Physiol*. 2007;292:L278-86.

97. Devereux G, Macdonald H, Hawrylowicz C. Vitamin D and asthma: time for intervention? *Am J Respir Crit Care Med*. 2009;179:739-40.

98. Sutherland ER, Goleva E, Jackson LP, Stevens AD, Leung DY. Vitamin D levels, lung function, and steroid response in adult asthma. *Am J Respir Crit Care Med.* 2010;181: 699-704.

99. Xystrakis E, Kusumakar S, Boswell S, Peek E, Urry Z, Richards DF, et al. Reversing the defective induction of IL-10-secreting regulatory T cells in glucocorticoid-resistant asthma patients. *J Clin Invest.* 2006;116:146-55.

100. Hothersall E, McSharry C, Thomson NC. Potential therapeutic role for statins in respiratory disease. *Thorax.* 2006;61:729-34.

101. Kim DY, Ryu SY, Lim JE, Lee YS, Ro JY. Anti-inflammatory mechanism of simvastatin in mouse allergic asthma model. *Eur J Pharmacol.* 2007;557:76-86.

102. Chiba Y, Sato S, Misawa M. Inhibition of antigen-induced bronchial smooth muscle hyperresponsiveness by lovastatin in mice. *J Smooth Muscle Res.* 2008;44:123-8.

103. Imamura M, Okunishi K, Ohtsu H, Nakagome K, Harada H, Tanaka R, et al. Pravastatin attenuates allergic airway inflammation by suppressing antigen sensitisation, interleukin 17 production and antigen presentation in the lung. *Thorax.* 2009;64:44-9.

104. Chiba Y, Arima J, Sakai H, Misawa M. Lovastatin inhibits bronchial hyperresponsiveness by reducing RhoA signaling in rat allergic asthma. *Am J Physiol Lung Cell Mol Physiol.* 2008;294:L705-13.

105. McKay A, Leung BP, McInnes IB, Thomson NC, Liew FY. A novel anti-inflammatory role of simvastatin in a murine model of allergic asthma. *J Immunol.* 2004;172:2903-8.

106. Zeki AA, Franzi L, Last J, Kenyon NJ. Simvastatin inhibits airway hyperreactivity: implications for the mevalonate pathway and beyond. *Am J Respir Crit Care Med.* 2009;180: 731-40.

107. Menzies D, Nair A, Meldrum KT, Fleming D, Barnes M, Lipworth BJ. Simvastatin does not exhibit therapeutic anti-inflammatory effects in asthma. *J Allergy Clin Immunol.* 2007;119:328-35.

108. Hothersall EJ, Chaudhuri R, McSharry C, Donnelly I, Lafferty J, McMahon AD, et al. Effects of atorvastatin added to inhaled corticosteroids on lung function and sputum cell counts in atopic asthma. *Thorax.* 2008;63:1070-5.

109. Cowan DC, Cowan JO, Palmay R, Williamson A, Taylor DR. Simvastatin in the treatment of asthma: lack of steroid-sparing effect. *Thorax.* 2010;65:891-6.

110. Braganza G, Chaudhuri R, McSharry C, Weir CJ, Donnelly I, Jolly L, et al. Effects of short-term treatment with atorvastatin in smokers with asthma—a randomized controlled trial. *BMC Pulm Med.* 2011;11:16.

111. Cox PG, Miller J, Mitzner W, Leff AR. Radiofrequency ablation of airway smooth muscle for sustained treatment of asthma: preliminary investigations. *Eur Respir J.* 2004;24: 659-63.

112. Danek CJ, Lombard CM, Dungworth DL, Cox PG, Miller JD, Biggs MJ, et al. Reduction in airway hyperresponsiveness to methacholine by the application of RF energy in dogs. *J Appl Physiol.* 2004;97:1946-53.

113. Brown RH, Wizeman W, Danek C, Mitzner W. In vivo evaluation of the effectiveness of bronchial thermoplasty with computed tomography. *J Appl Physiol.* 2005;98:1603-6.

114. Brown RH, Wizeman W, Danek C, Mitzner W. Effect of bronchial thermoplasty on airway distensibility. *Eur Respir J.* 2005;26:277-82.

115. Mayse M, Laviolette M, Rubin AS, et al. Clinical pearls for bronchial thermoplasty. *J Bronchol.* 2007;14:115-23.

116. Cox G, Miller JD, McWilliams A, Fitzgerald JM, Lam S. Bronchial thermoplasty for asthma. *Am J Respir Crit Care Med.* 2006;173:965-9.

117. Cox G, Thomson NC, Rubin AS, Niven RM, Corris PA, Siersted HC, et al. Asthma control during the year after bronchial thermoplasty. *N Engl J Med.* 2007;356:1327-37.

118. Pavord ID, Cox G, Thomson NC, Rubin AS, Corris PA, Niven RM, et al. Safety and efficacy of bronchial thermoplasty in symptomatic, severe asthma. *Am J Respir Crit Care Med.* 2007;176:1185-91.

119. Castro M, Rubin AS, Laviolette M, Fiterman J, De Andrade Lima M, Shah PL, et al. Effectiveness and safety of bronchial thermoplasty in the treatment of severe asthma: a multicenter, randomized, double-blind, sham-controlled clinical trial. *Am J Respir Crit Care Med.* 2010;181:116-24.

120. Thomson NC, Rubin AS, Niven RM, Corris PA, Siersted HC, Olivenstein R, et al. Long term (5 year) safety of bronchial thermoplasty: Asthma Intervention Research (AIR) trial. *BMC Pulm Med.* 2011;11:8.

121. Cox G, Miller JD, Goodwin S, FitzGerald JM, Hui L, Lam S. Long-term follow-up of bronchial thermoplasty for asthma: safety results at 5 years. *Am J Respir Crit Care Med.* 2008;177:A567.

122. Abramson MJ, Puy RM, Weiner JM. Injection allergen immunotherapy for asthma. *Cochrane Database Syst Rev.* 2010:CD001186.

123. Cox L, Nelson H, Lockey R, Calabria C, Chacko T, Finegold I, et al. Allergen immunotherapy: a practice parameter third update. *J Allergy Clin Immunol.* 2011;127:S1-S55.

124. Casale TB, Stokes JR. Future forms of immunotherapy. *J Allergy Clin Immunol.* 2011;127: 8-15.

125. Massanari M, Nelson H, Casale T, Busse W, Kianifard F, Geba GP, et al. Effect of pretreatment with omalizumab on the tolerability of specific immunotherapy in allergic asthma. *J Allergy Clin Immunol.* 2010;125:383-9.

126. Gøtzsche PC, Johansen HK. House dust mite control measures for asthma. *Cochrane Database Syst Rev.* 2008:CD001187.

127. Kilburn S, Lasserson TJ, McKean M. Pet allergen control measures for allergic asthma in children and adults. *Cochrane Database Syst Rev.* 2003:CD002989.

128. Wright GR, Howieson S, McSharry C, McMahon AD, Chaudhuri R, Thompson J, et al. Effect of improved home ventilation on asthma control and house dust mite allergen levels. *Allergy.* 2009;64:1671-80.

129. Wenzel SE. Asthma: defining of the persistent adult phenotypes. *Lancet.* 2006;368:804-13.

130. Thomson NC, Chaudhuri R. Identification and management of adults with asthma prone to exacerbations: can we do better? *BMC Pulm Med.* 2008;8:27.

131. Barnes PJ. Corticosteroid resistance in airway disease. *Proc Am Thorac Soc.* 2004;1:264-8.

132. Thomson NC, Chaudhuri R. Asthma in smokers: challenges and opportunities. *Curr Opin Pulm Med.* 2009;15:39-45.

133. Thomson NC, Spears M. The Role of Cigarette Smoking on Persistent Airflow Obstruction in Asthma. *Ann Respir Med.* 2010.

134. ten Brinke A, Zwinderman AH, Sterk PJ, Rabe KF, Bel EH. Factors associated with persistent airflow limitation in severe asthma. *Am J Respir Crit Care Med.* 2001;164:744-8.

135. Lee JH, Haselkorn T, Borish L, Rasouliyan L, Chipps BE, Wenzel SE. Risk factors associated with persistent airflow limitation in severe or difficult-to-treat asthma: insights from the TENOR study. *Chest.* 2007;132:1882-9.

136. Gupta S, Siddiqui S, Haldar P, Raj JV, Entwisle JJ, Wardlaw AJ, et al. Qualitative analysis of high-resolution CT scans in severe asthma. *Chest.* 2009;136:1521-8.

137. Hall IP, Sayers I. Pharmacogenetics and asthma: false hope or new dawn? *Eur Respir J.* 2007;29:1239-45.

138. Lima JJ, Blake KV, Tantisira KG, Weiss ST. Pharmacogenetics of asthma. *Curr Opin Pulm Med.* 2009;15:57-62.

139. Drazen JM, Yandava CN, Dubé L, Szczerback N, Hippensteel R, Pillari A, et al. Pharmaco-genetic association between ALOX5 promoter genotype and the response to anti-asthma treatment. *Nat Genet.* 1999;22:168-70.

140. Lima JJ, Zhang S, Grant A, Shao L, Tantisira KG, Allayee H, et al. Influence of leukotriene pathway polymorphisms on response to montelukast in asthma. *Am J Respir Crit Care Med.* 2006;173:379-85.

141. Klotsman M, York TP, Pillai SG, Vargas-Irwin C, Sharma SS, van den Oord EJ, et al. Pharmacogenetics of the 5-lipoxygenase biosynthetic pathway and variable clinical response to montelukast. *Pharmacogenet Genomics.* 2007;17:189-96.

142. Sampson AP, Siddiqui S, Buchanan D, Howarth PH, Holgate ST, Holloway JW, et al. Variant LTC(4) synthase allele modifies cysteinyl leukotriene synthesis in eosinophils and predicts clinical response to zafirlukast. *Thorax.* 2000;55:S28-31.

143. Currie GP, Lima JJ, Sylvester JE, Lee DK, Cockburn WJ, Lipworth BJ. Leukotriene C4 synthase polymorphisms and responsiveness to leukotriene antagonists in asthma. *Br J Clin Pharmacol.* 2003;56:422-6.

144. Tantisira KG, Hwang ES, Raby BA, Silverman ES, Lake SL, Richter BG, et al. TBX21: a functional variant predicts improvement in asthma with the use of inhaled cortico-steroids. *Proc Natl Acad Sci U S A.* 2004;101:18099-104.

145. Tantisira KG, Lake S, Silverman ES, Palmer LJ, Lazarus R, Silverman EK, et al. Cortico-steroid pharmacogenetics: association of sequence variants in CRHR1 with improved lung function in asthmatics treated with inhaled corticosteroids. *Hum Mol Genet.* 2004;13:1353-9.

146. Tantisira KG, Silverman ES, Mariani TJ, Xu J, Richter BG, Klanderman BJ, et al. FCER2: a pharmacogenetic basis for severe exacerbations in children with asthma. *J Allergy Clin Immunol.* 2007;120:1285-91.

147. Haldar P, Pavord ID. Noneosinophilic asthma: a distinct clinical and pathologic pheno-type. *J Allergy Clin Immunol.* 2007;119:1043-52.

148. Simpson JL, Scott R, Boyle MJ, Gibson PG. Inflammatory subtypes in asthma: assessment and identification using induced sputum. *Respirology.* 2006;11:54-61.

149. Woodruff PG, Modrek B, Choy DF, Jia G, Abbas AR, Ellwanger A, et al. T-helper type 2-driven inflammation defines major subphenotypes of asthma. *Am J Respir Crit Care Med.* 2009;180:388-95.

Index

Please note page numbers with *f* and *t* indicate figure and table, respectively.